# THE NATURAL WAY SERIES

Increasing numbers of people worldwide are falling victim to illnesses which modern medicine, for all its technical advances, seems often powerless to prevent – and sometimes actually causes. To find cures for these so-called 'diseases of civilization' more and more people are turning to 'natural' medicine for an answer. The *Natural Way* series aims to offer clear, practical and reliable guidance to the safest, gentlest and most effective treatments available – and so to give sufferers and their families the information they need to make their own choices about the most suitable treatments.

*Other titles in the* Natural Way *series*

# THE NATURAL WAY
# Multiple Sclerosis

*Richard Thomas*

*Series editor*
*Richard Thomas*

*Series medical consultants*
*Dr Peter Albright MD & Dr David Peters MD*

Approved by the
AMERICAN HOLISTIC MEDICAL ASSOCIATION
& BRITISH HOLISTIC MEDICAL ASSOCIATION

# ELEMENT
Shaftesbury, Dorset ● Rockport, Massachusetts
Brisbane, Queensland

© Element Books Limited 1995

First published in Great Britain in 1995 by
Element Books Limited
Shaftesbury, Dorset, SP7 8BP

Published in the USA in 1995 by
Element Books, Inc.
PO Box 830, Rockport, MA 01966

Published in Australia in 1995 by
Element Books Limited
for Jacaranda Wiley Limited
33 Park Road, Milton, Brisbane 4064

Cover design by Max Fairbrother
Text illustrations by David Woodroffe
Designed and typeset by Linda Reed and Joss Nizan
Printed and bound in Great Britain by
BPC Paperbacks Ltd

British Library Cataloguing in Publication
data available

Library of Congress Cataloging in Publication
data available

ISBN 1–85230–715–3

# Contents

# Illustrations

For Jane and Liz

# Acknowledgements

My very great and grateful thanks go to the many people with MS who so generously and good-humouredly gave me time and information about themselves and others; to the many therapists and doctors who helped in the same way, particularly Professor Ian McDonald, Professor Alastair Compston, Dr Patrick Kingsley, Dr Bob Lawrence, Susie Cornell and Vicky Mainprize; to the International Federation of Multiple Sclerosis Societies, the Multiple Sclerosis Society of Great Britain and Northern Ireland, the MS Society of New South Wales (Australia), the Federation of Multiple Sclerosis Therapy Centres, the Multiple Sclerosis Training, Education & Research Trust; to the series' omniscient consultants Dr Peter Albright and Dr David Peters; and especially to the writer and broadcaster Judy Graham, an MS sufferer whose skilful help and intelligent guidance on the correct path to tread for the greatest benefit for all, away from vested interests, proved invaluable.

# Introduction

Multiple sclerosis (MS) is one of the commonest diseases of the central nervous system. Distressing and frightening, it presently affects about 2.5 million people worldwide – including some 250,000 in North America, 90,000 in the UK and 40,000 in Australia and New Zealand.

MS is a presently incurable and potentially life-threatening disease of unknown origin that can disable and cripple those unfortunate enough to suffer from it. Roughly one in every 1,000 people could get it and about one in 20,000 do. It can start at almost any age and affect any part of the body.

Well-known sufferers include the comedian Richard Pryor, model Vivien Neves, film director Bryan Forbes, radio presenter Stuart Henry, pop singers Clifford T Ward and Ronnie Lane, TV weatherman Bernard Davey, and writer and broadcaster Judy Graham. Past sufferers have included the film actress Margaret Leighton and cellist Jacqueline du Pré.

Though incurable at the moment, a number of safe, gentle and effective treatments are available that have all been shown to help certain people some of the time. These treatments include dietary therapy and nutrition, exercise and yoga, massage and aromatherapy, acupuncture, oxygen therapies, psychotherapy and counselling, hydrotherapy, reflexology and homoeopathy.

Conventional medicine, by contrast, generally has a much narrower approach to the disease, concentrating largely on 'management drugs' like steroids and drugs that control the body's defence system. Though it can be successful in dealing with byproducts such as urinary tract infection, conventional medicine still feels largely helpless in the face of MS.

The lesson of the few people who have pioneered a range of treatments for MS that do not rely on drugs is that much can be done. And you don't have to wait for others. Indeed, the earlier you start helping yourself, the more likely you are to reap benefits.

This book sets out to help you trace the treatment or therapy (and therapist for that matter) most likely to help you. It says that everyone can be helped to some degree. It doesn't claim to know all the answers or to be infallible but it does give you the choice. One thing is for sure: you won't know unless you try.

# CHAPTER 1

# What is multiple sclerosis?

*How and why it develops and who it affects*

Multiple sclerosis, or MS for short, is one of the commonest diseases of the central nervous system. According to all official information on the subject, it strikes at random, often causing paralysis and affecting sight and speech – and is incurable.

The basic cause of this tragic and still quite baffling illness is a mystery. It happens because of damage to the thin protective layer of fatty membrane, called the *myelin sheath*, that surrounds the nerve tracts in the brain and, more especially, the spinal cord.

Myelin sheath acts like the insulation around electrical wires. It allows the current – or in the case of the human body the electrical signals – to travel through without loss of power or strength. Any damage to this protective layer can cause the electrical signals to 'leak' and so lose power and become distorted.

In MS this damage is the result of inflammation. The inflammation makes the sheath lose some of its covering – a process known as *demyelination*. Hard scar tissue then forms over these damaged patches or *lesions* and this is what gives MS its name. 'Multiple sclerosis' (or, sometimes, 'disseminated sclerosis') means literally 'multiple scarring or hardening' – sclerosis being from a Greek word meaning hard or tough.

As the central nervous system controls the whole body, patches of demyelination, or *plaques* as the doctors call them, can occur anywhere. Symptoms can come and go and this is why the disease is commonly described as a 'relapsing–remitting disease'.

What controls relapses and remissions and how they occur remains one of the many mysteries of this complex disease that the experts are trying to solve.

### How myelin sheath damage causes MS

As *figure 1* shows, scarring of the myelin sheath damages nerves directly. This damage causes distorted or wrong signals to go to the muscles via the brain – and so the muscles don't work, or don't work properly.

Dymyelination can happen anywhere in the central nervous system but the parts most usually affected are the nerve to the eyes (*optic nerve*), brain, brain stem and spinal cord. More about how nerves and muscles work will be found in *Chapter 2*.

### Symptoms of MS

Symptoms resulting from the onset of MS are as wide and varied as there are people, depending not just on the nerves affected and the parts of the body they serve but the particular constitution and makeup of the individual affected. There is simply no set pattern.

MS symptoms can include any or all of the following (those most commonly felt) but may not be on this list at all. One person started with blinding headaches. Equally, symptoms may come and go, even within a day, varying in intensity, and switch from one part of the body to another, depending on which nerves are affected (see *Chapter 2*).

For example nerves responsible for making muscles

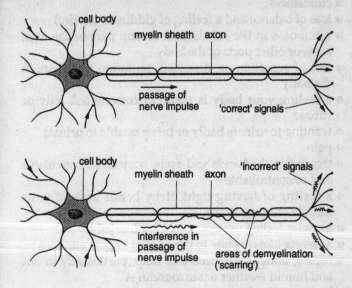

**Fig. 1 A healthy nerve (top) and a damaged nerve in someone with MS (bottom)**
By courtesy of the MS Society of Great Britain & Northern Ireland

work (*motor nerves*) can cause problems with walking, using your hands or swallowing, while nerves that control bodily sensations such as touch or sight (*sensory nerves*) can affect sight and cause numbness, tingling and pain.

The most often reported symptoms of MS, in some order of how commonly they occur, are:

- double, blurred or loss of vision in one or both eyes
- tingling or a 'pins and needles' feeling
- slurred speech
- difficulty in walking
- dragging either foot
- loss of coordination

- clumsiness
- loss of balance and a feeling of giddiness (*vertigo*)
- numbness in the hands, feet or any part of the legs, arms or other parts of the body
- loss of sensation or 'distorted' sensation anywhere in the body
- a feeling your body is made of cottonwool, jelly or rubber
- wanting to urinate badly or being unable to urinate
- pain
- tremors in the hands and arms, sometimes convulsive and uncontrollable
- a feeling of having tight, itchy bands around your middle or lower limbs
- muscles feeling useless (*spastic*) or like jelly
- a feeling like frostbite in the ends of fingers and toes
- feeling unnaturally tired and limp, particularly in hot and humid weather or surroundings
- having difficulty concentrating or remembering things
- feeling depressed for no particular reason

*Note* Having these symptoms is no more a guarantee you have MS than a lack of them guarantees you don't. Some are serious and others mild. It must be emphasized that MS remains an immensely complex and puzzling condition no one fully understands yet, but your chances of having MS are highest if your symptoms are in the top end of the above list.

## What happens in MS

Apart from lack of coordination and slurred speech – leading to some people mistakenly thinking someone with MS is drunk or mentally deficient – damage to the central nervous system can typically also cause the following 'side-effects'.

- *Fatigue* In MS this is not the same as general tiredness and muscle ache and seems to be something quite definite but subtle that a sufferer feels but cannot adequately describe, a doctor cannot detect and the cause of which is unknown.
- *Incontinence* Bladder and bowels are controlled by the nervous system so demyelination can commonly cause people with MS to want to go to the toilet very quickly or frequently or both.
- *Mental and emotional problems* People with MS can suffer problems with memory and concentration and often find it hard to control emotions, crying or laughing for no obvious reason.
- *Speech and language problems* Distorted nerve signals in the brain can also cause speech and language difficulties in about half of all sufferers.
- *Sexual problems* Men can find it difficult getting and keeping an erection and ejaculating while women can suffer from a dry vagina and lack of clitoral excitement.

## Who is most at risk, and why

- For reasons not yet fully understood MS affects women more than men. The ratio is about 3:2 – that is, three women are affected for every two men.
- Age is also a factor. MS is rarely seen in pre-teenage children and rarely starts in people over 65. The average age of onset is mid-20s to mid-30s, with roughly 60 per cent between 15 and 35.
- There does seem to be 'an inherited tendency' (or 'predisposition') to MS. That means 'MS genes' can be passed on. Recent research has shown around 66 per cent of sufferers have 'MS genes' and the chances of getting MS go up hugely – from a lifetime risk of one in 800 to one in 50 – if a parent has MS.

- Climate and environment also seem to be a major factor. MS is far more common in countries with a temperate climate, such as Europe and parts of North America, than in tropical areas.

Unfortunately the reasons for these anomalies of sex and location remain a mystery, though various theories have been put forward. Other theories why some people get MS and others don't include dietary deficiencies, problems with the way the body processes certain chemicals, a defect in the body's natural defence mechanism,

---

### The inheritance factor

Can MS be inherited? The latest evidence is that it probably can be in a sense – although not in the same way that someone inherits a disease like the blood disorder *haemophilia* for example. One of the cases described in *chapter 7* is of a young woman with MS whose father also has MS.

What it amounts to is that people with 'MS genes' are probably more likely to get MS than those without – but it does not mean they are bound to get it. Researchers in Australia concluded after a nationwide survey of MS in 1988 that genetic susceptibility played little part in the geographical differences there, saying that their findings 'argued strongly for the existence of an important environmental factor in MS'.

Work in Britain and Canada nevertheless seems to be confirming the idea of an inherited susceptibility as a result of 'MS genes' in genetic makeup. An international database is in the process of being set up as a result of this research that hopes to establish a 'gene profile' of people with MS.

The database is a joint UK–Canadian venture between Professor Alistair Compston, of Addenbrooke's Hospital, Cambridge, UK, and Professor George Ebers, of University Hospital, London, Ontario, Canada. But it is expected to be some time yet before it is ready.

'poisoning' from mercury amalgam fillings, environmental pollution, and childhood infection.

These are described in more detail in *chapter 3*. But what we do know is that MS is *not* infectious or contagious – you can't catch it like a cold or chicken pox from someone who has it – and it is *not* a mental disorder or 'nerves' of the sort needing psychiatric treatment (though MS can have profound psychological effects at every stage of the disease – see *Chapter 8*).

## The types of MS

MS is a complex condition and frequently no two people experience the same thing. In fact it is often said that each of the 2.5 million sufferers in the world will tell a different story. In other words, each has their own unique type of MS. That's what makes it particularly difficult for doctors to diagnose in the first place. There have even been stories of some people diagnosed with MS who were subsequently found not to have MS at all, and vice versa.

The UK Office of Health Economics has defined seven different types of MS but most experts generally now agree on four main types. In order of increasing seriousness they are:

- *Benign* Some 20 per cent of sufferers have a benign form of MS in which disability is minimal, even after many years. Deterioration is still possible, though, in spite of the disease remaining inactive for many years.
- *Relapsing–remitting* (or *chronic relapsing*) This is the most common and unpredictable form of MS, with 60 per cent falling into this category. Symptoms come and go, affecting different parts of the body with varying severity. Patients often recover from attacks at first but there is usually a gradual worsening over time.

- *Chronic progressive* Around 10 per cent of sufferers have this form of MS – where there is a slow but steady deterioration with no clear attacks or remissions.
- *Rapidly deteriorating* or *galloping* This is the most serious form of the disease, affecting around 10 per cent of cases, and is the result of widespread demyelination of the nerves in the brain. The MS takes a 'galloping' form and can be fatal in around five to ten years.

---

**Patient profile**

A large practice in a small town in southern England has the following typical profile of patients with MS:

| | Benign | Relapsing –remitting | Progressive | Galloping | Total |
|---|---|---|---|---|---|
| Women | 4 | 6 | 2 | nil | 12 |
| Men | 2 | 3 | nil | 1 | 6 |
| **Total** | **6** | **9** | **2** | **1** | **18** |

**Case 1**

Sally, a 35-year-old nurse, was diagnosed with MS at 27 after three attacks coinciding with her three pregnancies. Her symptoms are mainly right-sided and come and go. In 1995 she was almost symptom-free and well enough to be still working as a nurse.

**Case 2**

Sandra, 55, was diagnosed at 43 after symptoms starting four years earlier of blurred vision in one eye, calf cramps, frequent falls and a burning feeling at the base of her spine. She had no remissions and within two years was wheelchair-bound. By 1995 she had had to move to a flat for the disabled requiring daily care from her husband and district nurses.

---

## MS and life expectancy

Despite what many people think, MS does not greatly affect life expectancy in most cases. Except in those small percentage of cases of 'galloping MS', the disease is not what doctors call a 'terminal illness'. Though mobility is usually affected towards the end of a sufferer's life only one in five need a wheelchair.

In severe cases infection in the chest or urinary tract can set in that can lead to death – and both are a common cause of death in people with severe MS. But the condition normally has to be extremely severe for this sort of complication to occur and most people with MS do not die prematurely these days.

The significant thing seems to be what happens to you in the first five years of developing the condition. If you do not get noticeably worse in that time doctors consider you have a fairly good 'prognosis' – that is, your chances of not getting too seriously ill and of living out a reasonably normal life are good.

In the next chapter we look in more detail at the nervous system.

# CHAPTER 2

# All about the nervous and immune systems

*What they are and how they work*

MS is basically a disease of the body's central nervous system – the brain and spinal cord. Damage to the nerves in the brain and spinal cord means the right signals do not reach the various parts of the body and the right signals are not sent back. To see how this happens let's look at how the body's nervous system works in more detail.

### The nervous system

Nerves are the key to a biological understanding of MS. Nerves are complex fibres interlacing the human body like wiring in a house. This network of nerves is known as the *nervous system* (*see figure 2*) and it conducts electrical impulses that are created in the body chemically. The nervous system is really three systems:

- the *motor nervous system*, controlling the muscles
- the *sensory nervous system*, controlling information from the five main bodily senses of sight, sound, touch, taste and smell to the brain
- the *autonomic nervous system*, controlling automatic functions such as breathing, heartbeat and digestion

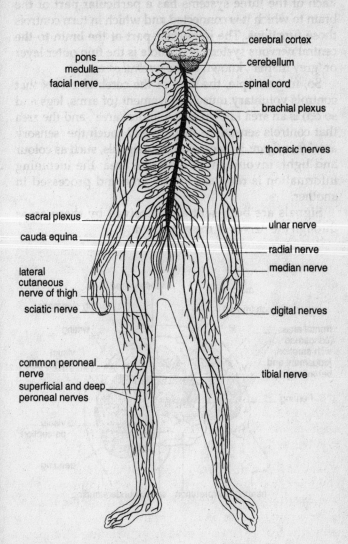

**Fig. 2  The nervous system**

Each of the three systems has a particular part of the brain to which it is connected and which in turn controls those functions. The important part of the brain to the central nervous system as a whole is the thin outer layer or 'grey matter', known as the *cerebral cortex*.

So, for example, the area of the cerebral cortex that controls voluntary muscle movement (of arms, legs and so on) is an area known as the 'motor area', and the area that controls sensations of pain and touch the 'sensory area' (see *figure 3*). More complex signals, such as colour and light, involve more than one area: the incoming information is received in one area and processed in another.

Signals are both sent and received by these areas through the nerves of the *spinal cord*.

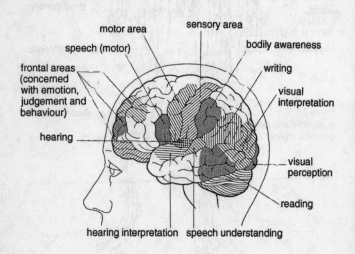

**Fig. 3 The 'function areas' of the brain**

## The spinal cord and its nerves

The spinal cord is a thick 'cord' of nerve fibre that runs down the hollow tunnel through the middle of the bones of the spine and is rather like the mains cable bringing the supply of electricity into a house. Signals from the brain are relayed via nerves down the spinal cord and from there to every part of the body and back again.

The nerves radiating out from the spinal cord are known as *spinal nerves* and are some of the most important in the body. Spinal nerves consist of a number of nerve fibres bundled together in groups, so a single spinal nerve contains hundreds of individual nerve fibres (see *figure 4*).

The electrochemical signals that travel through nerve fibres go along a long central extension of a nerve cell known as an *axon*. Axons are the equivalent of the copper wire in electricity cables and, like cables, they are encased and protected by an outer layer that acts as both

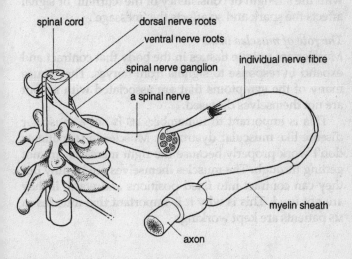

Fig. 4  How nerves connect to the spinal cord

insulation and conductor. It is this outer layer that is the all-important *myelin sheath*.

Spinal nerves carry messages to and from the spinal cord from both the motor and sensory nervous systems. These messages pass through a switching process in the spinal cord before they arrive at the part of the brain controlling the right response.

So, for example, if the sensory nerves in the hand pick up a sensation of heat and pain from touching a hot saucepan, that is then relayed via the spinal nerves and spinal cord to the sensory area of the brain. The sensory area sends a signal to the neighbouring motor area and that area transmits a signal back via the spinal cord and nerves that tells the muscles of the hand to drop or let go of the saucepan quickly.

'Messages' are passed from one cell to another (across gaps called *synapses*) purely electrically, rather like a spark crossing between two contacts. Any interference with the strength or consistency of the 'current' or signal affects the spark and so affects the 'message'.

### The role of muscles in MS

Muscles are unique tissues in the body that contract and expand in response to signals from nerves. They cause many of the symptoms that are associated with MS but are not themselves diseased.

This is important to remember. MS is not a muscular disease like muscular dystrophy. Muscles in MS patients don't work properly because the right messages are not getting through. The muscles themselves are healthy but they can contract into fixed positions and waste if they are not used. This is why it is important that muscles in MS patients are kept working.

## The immune system

Though no one really knows yet what causes MS (see *chapter 3*) there is general agreement among most experts that the body's defence system or *immune system* is involved in various ways.

The immune system is the mechanism the body has for fighting threats to your health. In a normally healthy person it is at work the whole time. Like an army of soldiers it is on constant watch defending you against anything that might hurt or harm you.

In MS the immune system seems to be defective, turning against the body instead of supporting it. This is what is meant when doctors call it an *auto-immune disease*. Examples include allergies (where the immune system over-reacts to normally harmless substances such as animal hair or pollen) and Aids. MS may be another. But what is the immune system supposed to do and how does it do it?

For something so important, your body's immune system is deceptively simple. It consists basically of your blood supply and small sets of organs called the *tonsils*, *thymus gland*, *lymph nodes* and *spleen* (see *figure 5*).

Defence against disease is essentially a function of the white cells in blood and it is one of the jobs of this group of organs to produce these white cells, known as *leucocytes*. (Some white cells are also made in bone marrow which produces the blood's supply of red cells; see *box on page 19*.)

White blood cells produce substances which defend the body against attack from anything harmful such as a virus. These defending substances are known as *antibodies* (attacking substances are known as *antigens*). Antibodies are made by particular sorts of white blood cells known as *lymphocytes* and they come in five types, called *immunoglobulins*, each with a different function.

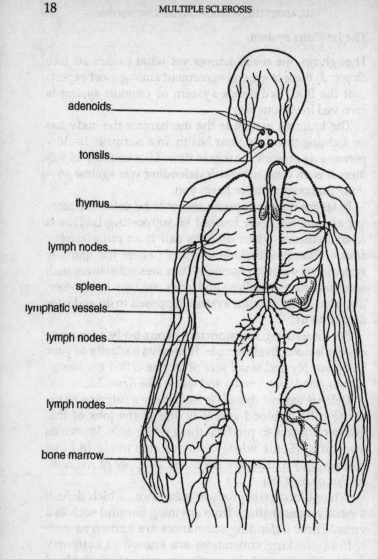

adenoids

tonsils

thymus

lymph nodes

spleen

lymphatic vessels

lymph nodes

lymph nodes

bone marrow

**Fig. 5  The immune system**

## How blood fights infection

The blood in our bodies is made up of roughly

- 40% red cells (known as *erythrocytes*)
- 60% plasma, a semi-clear mixture of proteins (including vitamins) and mineral salts
- a very small amount is made up of white cells (*leucocytes*) and special clotting agents called *platelets*
- other ingredients include the *hormones,* chemicals controlling the body's essential activities

Blood is made mainly in bone marrow (especially the long bones of the ribs, backbone, breastbone and skull) but also in the lymph nodes and spleen. All red blood cells and some white cells come from bone marrow but white cells are also produced by the lymph nodes and the spleen.

White cells (*leucocytes*) come in three main types:

- *macrophages*
- bone-marrow cells (known as *B-cells*)
- thymus cells (*T-cells*)

*Macrophages* are large cells (seen through a miscroscope they are a mixture of round and elongated shapes) and are the major fighting cells. They are the 'cleaners-up'. They surround and 'hoover up' not only any harmful substance such as a virus (the general term used by doctors is *antigen*) but also the defending substance (known as an *antibody*) before disposing of everything through the *lymphatic system*.

*B-cells* make antibodies that destroy antigens. They also have a memory that can recognize and attack past viruses.

*T-cells* are split into 'T-helpers' and 'T-suppressors' and both are needed to keep the immune response balanced. T-cells contain *cytotoxins* that kill infected cells and make a virus-blocking protein called *interferon*.

## Summary

If the nervous system is the body's 'telecommunications system', relaying messages to and fro between the brain and the muscles via the spinal cord, the immune system can be seen as part of the 'maintenance department', keeping the equipment in good repair.

Unfortunately in today's world any number of things, from the air we breathe to the state of our emotions, can affect or interfere with the immune system so that it doesn't work as well as it should and keep the equipment in as good repair as it should.

Faults with both the nervous and immune systems lead to MS and we'll look at the causes of those next.

# CHAPTER 3

# Causes and risk factors in MS

*What they are and how they affect you*

What causes MS is still a mystery. We know that the *immediate* cause is damage to the protective myelin coating around the nerves in the central nervous system and that this damage is caused by inflammation.

The most widely-held medical view is that this inflammation is caused by the body itself. Most doctors believe it is the body turning against itself that is the problem. They think that particular blood cells called *T-helper cells* enter the central nervous system and inflame the myelin, but what causes them to do this is now the key question for researchers worldwide.

## Possible causes of MS

MS is what doctors call a 'multi-factorial disease'. That means they believe any number of factors may lie behind it and drawing up a neat hierarchy of cause-and-effect has not so far been possible.

Among various theories and ideas of what causes MS the leading contenders so far are:

- heavy metal poisoning
- eating too many saturated fats
- low levels of essential fatty acids
- food allergies
- childhood infections

- carbon monoxide and environmental poisoning
- low-level radiation
- prolonged use of the contraceptive pill
- severe emotional trauma and stress
- physical injury
- vaccinations
- overuse of antibiotics
- genetic predisposition
- climate and geography

*Heavy metal poisoning*

Substances in the blood harmful to nerves are kept separate by a special filtering layer in the walls of blood vessels called the *endothelium*. This is particularly important in the brain where the filter mechanism is known as the 'blood–brain barrier'.

Any number of events can cause this barrier to be breached, including stress, tiredness, fever, emotional upset, heat, injury and eating too much fat (see *below*). This allows chemicals from the blood poisonous to the nervous system into the brain where they can cause serious damage. Heavy metals such as mercury, cadmium and aluminium are well known examples of such potent *neurotoxins*.

Some researchers now believe that MS is a direct result of neurotoxins from the blood entering the central nervous system through the brain.

Swedish researchers, for example, claim they have found mercury levels more than seven times higher than normal in the spinal fluid of people with MS. They blame particularly the high amounts of mercury used in routine dental fillings (known as 'amalgams') and Sweden is now leading the world in banning the use of mercury in fillings.

*Eating too many saturated fats*

Professor Roy Swank, American champion since 1948 of

the low-fat diet for MS, and Dr Philip James, British champion of the use of high pressure or *hyperbaric* oxygen, both also believe it is the breach of the blood–brain barrier that plays a central role in MS.

Professor Swank, head of neurology at Oregon Health Sciences University, was the first to notice that MS was only found in those parts of the world where a lot of saturated fat was eaten. Too much saturated fat, he believes, damages the walls of the blood vessels allowing toxins to leak into the nervous system through the brain (see *above*).

Dr James, on the other hand, believes MS is caused by fat *embolism* (blockage) in the blood vessels as a result of the body's mishandling of saturated fats.

Saturated fats are found in foods such as animal fat (meat, lard, dripping), butter, milk, cream, cheese, margarine, batter, blended vegetable oils, coconut oil, salad cream and ice cream.

## Low levels of essential fatty acids

British researcher Professor RHS Thompson first suggested in the 1960s that MS may be caused by a problem the body has in handling unsaturated fats properly, particularly those called *essential fatty acids* (EFAs).

Professor Thomson found people with MS lacked two particular EFAs known as *linoleic acid* and *arachidonic acid* in their cells. This defect, called 'Thompson's anomaly', means the cell membranes in the body of a person with MS are weak and not working as they should. Later researchers have confirmed this in work with blood cells.

## Food allergies

The link between food and illness is still controversial amongst most doctors but a growing number are starting to take it seriously. The word commonly used is 'allergy'.

A food allergy is when certain foods cause specific symptoms of ill-health. In other words, the body reacts to the food (which is a nothing more than a collection of chemicals) as if it were a poison of some sort. Doctors say that what is happening is, strictly speaking, an 'intolerance' to that food.

An American neurologist, Dr Robert Soll, was among the first to link food intolerance to MS after noting that many sufferers 'frequently display a profile of numerous allergies.' He believed that MS is the end result of the body of susceptible people absorbing *endotoxins* – bacterial poisons produced by an infection – into the bloodstream through the intestines.

### Childhood infections

Many leading researchers think infections in childhood from viruses or bacteria are the most likely explanations for what triggers MS. The theory is that the virus or bacterium does not clear the system but lies dormant, weakening the immune system and causing MS in those with a genetic weakness for it.

### Viruses

Possible culprits include:

- flu
- glandular fever (or *infectious mononucleosis*), caused by the *Epstein-Barr* virus.
- *hepatitis* (a viral infection of the liver)
- viral *pneumonia* (inflammation of the lungs)
- shingles (*Herpes zoster*)

The shingles virus is the same virus that causes chicken pox. Dr Patrick Kingsley, a British doctor who specializes in MS, claims to have successfully helped some 3,000 sufferers in 15 years by removing the shingles virus homoeopathically – though there has been no independent confirmation of this so far.

Though MS researchers have been trying unsuccessfully for years to find evidence of a virus still in the body as a cause of MS, this theory is still a firm favourite among sufferers themselves. Some 47 per cent of sufferers surveyed in Southampton, southern England, believed their MS had been caused by the delayed effects of a childhood illness coupled with stress.

## Bacteria

Researchers have found that *sinusitis*, inflammation of the sinuses, is 17 times more common in people with MS than others and this means the *streptococcus* bacterium may be involved somehow.

There are a number of streptococci and they commonly cause throat infections – 'strep throat' – particularly in childhood. They can also lead to more serious conditions such as *tonsillitis*, *scarlet fever* and *quinsy*.

## Cardon monoxide and environmental poisoning

Laboratory tests in America have shown that carbon monoxide poisoning can cause myelin sheath damage and general degeneration of the central nervous system. So the theory is that carbon monoxide – which is the poisonous gas given off by car exhausts – may be to blame for MS because MS is common where traffic fumes are also high such as in North America and Europe.

This idea has led, in turn, to the suggestion that other forms of environmental pollution may equally be involved in MS, in particular in contributing to a decrease in immune system functioning and allowing toxins into the central nervous system.

## Low-level radiation

Many scientists now believe that even very low frequency radiation, such as that given off by high voltage power lines, radar, TV and computers can be extremely damaging to susceptible people. A British researcher, Dr

Jane Clarke, claimed in 1983 that MS was caused by just such radiation, including that from microwave ovens.

Extremely low frequency (ELF) radiation such as that used in microwave ovens heats things up from the inside out and so bypasses the body's normal heat receptors on the skin surface. Dr Clarke claimed that ELF radiation was damaging myelin sheath in susceptible people by overheating it in a way they would not have been aware.

She suggested that one of the reason sufferers might have been susceptible is because of a copper deficiency in their early diet that left the myelin sheath in their bodies abnormally thin to start with.

### The 'pill'

The champion of the theory that long-term use of the contraceptive pill is involved in MS is a British doctor, Ellen Grant. A specialist in female hormone disorders, Dr Grant claims the pill is the direct cause of the higher incidence of MS among women over men and this was predicted as long ago as 1969 in the prestigious *Journal of the American Medical Association*.

According to Dr Grant, author of *The Bitter Pill* (Corgi, UK, 1986) and *Sexual Chemistry* (Cedar, UK, 1994), prolonged use of *progesterone* – the main active hormone in the contraceptive pill – depresses the immune system by reducing the amount of antibodies produced by the body.

But her theory is dismissed by other doctors who say she has not produced enough strong evidence for the connection.

### Emotional trauma

Severe emotional trauma or stress – such as a bereavement, divorce, redundancy or moving house – are known to depress the immune system and, sometimes, cause the blood–brain barrier to be breached.

The combined effect is a potent trigger for many disease conditions and may be also in MS where some researchers have noted a connection between such events and MS (see *box below*).

## Physical injury

Damage to the spinal column as a result of whiplash injury, a bad fall or playing sport has been claimed to contribute indirectly to MS by creating 'weak spots' in the spinal cord that can be subsequently 'attacked', often many years later, by an infection – so aggravating symptoms of MS (see *box below*).

---

### A sufferer's research

In 1994 physical therapist and MS sufferer Susie Cornell completed a study of 80 people at her clinic in Chelmsford, south-east England, that she claims has identified five key factors as being behind MS:

- persistent throat infection throughout life, starting in childhood
- serious physical injury at some stage in life (eg car accident, sports injury, major fall)
- serious viral infection at some stage in life (eg pneumonia, glandular fever, hepatitis)
- serious emotional trauma at some stage in life (eg divorce, bereavement, redundancy)
- poor diet for a prolonged period

The study looked at two groups of 40 people, one with MS and the other without. Their past history showed:

| Incidence of | Group with MS | Group without MS |
|---|---|---|
| Throat infections | 75% | 25% |
| Physical injury | 75% | 25% |
| Viral infection | 70% | 30% |
| Emotional trauma | 60% | 40% |
| Poor diet | 60% | 40% |

---

## Vaccinations

Many MS sufferers have reported developing symptoms soon after having had a vaccination. Anti-flu vaccination has been often cited but others blamed have included immunization for overseas travel such as smallpox.

A few researchers in Britain and America, notably Dr Robert Mendelsohn, have subsequently pointed an accusing finger at routine immunization programmes as a cause of myelin sheath damage but no definitive evidence of this has so far emerged nor the mechanism by which it might occur.

## Overuse of antibiotics

Antibiotics are drugs that kill bacterial infection by destroying all bacteria in the body, good as well as bad. In the past they were frequently given for viral infections against which they are now known to be useless.

Overuse of antibiotics can result not only in a weakened immune system but, occasionally, a serious overgrowth of the yeast fungus *Candida albicans*. This can lead to the immunity-compromising condition known as *candidosis* or *candidiasis*.

An American doctor, William Crook, was the first to theorize about this, but most natural therapists are now aware of the yeast problem.

## Genetic predisposition

As explained in *Chapter 1* there is now growing evidence of a factor in some people's genes that makes them much more likely to get MS, particularly if a close relative or parent has MS. This is what is known as having a 'genetic predisposition'.

According to the latest research, over three times more people with MS have two particular genes – known as DW2 and DR2 – than normal. The genes are found in only about 20 per cent of the population at large but in 70 per cent of people with MS.

*Climate and geography*

Studies in Australia have shown that Tasmania, in the cold south, with a sixth of the population of Queensland, in the much hotter north, has *four times* the incidence of MS. In Tasmania it is about 75 per 100,000 people against just 11 per 100,000 in northern Queensland.

Experts are certain climate is involved in some way because people who move from tropical areas to temperate ones become just as susceptible to MS as people born and bred there. Why this should be no one is yet sure, though it may have something to do with temperature or diet or both.

### The latest theories

The very latest research suggests that the true story may be a mixture of inherently faulty myelin tissue and poor protection by a faulty or 'compromised' immune system. The picture is by no means certain yet but at least a number of factors have been identified that seem to suggest this latest idea is on the right track.

For example, research in America, Britain and New Zealand has confirmed that the mishandling of essential fatty acids means that *none* of the cells in an MS sufferer's body are built properly. Myelin tissue is probably then singled out because of the specific genetic makeup of people who get MS.

Other researchers, meanwhile, have confirmed that both white and red blood cells are not quite normal in MS sufferers. The predominant red cells seem to be elongated instead of circular, affecting the way blood flows, while the white cells – particularly those known as *T-helper cells* – have been shown to turn against myelin when they cross into the central nervous system. They then start to gobble myelin up instead of defending it as they are supposed to.

## What all this means for people with MS

The heartening thing for people with MS is that if this latest picture is the correct one then it explains why the many treatments and approaches in this book are able to help so many people – because faulty tissue and a faulty immune system can both be treated to some extent.

Not so long ago it was thought that once myelin tissue was damaged that was it. But it is now known this is not so: myelin can be regenerated. A British-based international research organization called the Myelin Project has been trying since 1990 to encourage research into finding ways myelin can be helped to grow again.

Writer and broadcaster Judy Graham, herself an MS sufferer, has made the point that although myelin is a relatively stable structure, individual components of it do turn over, with old components being broken down and replaced with new components.

The same is true of the immune system. A faulty immune system is a problem with a growing number of people of all ages and both sexes today, not just those with MS. This is largely, it is believed, because of the increasing stresses and strains of modern life coupled with unhealthy eating and living habits and the poor quality of our basic air and water. But it, too, can be repaired – or at least improved.

At the same time, changes in living and eating can not only strengthen body tissues but help reinforce the blood–brain barrier that seems to play such a significant role in the development of MS.

In the next chapter we'll see what you can do for yourself.

# CHAPTER 4

# How to help yourself

*Tips and guidelines for prevention and treatment*

People with MS are fortunate in one way. Because so little was done for sufferers in the past a large number of treatments have been tried out and tested by those not prepared to sit down and do nothing.

The result is that an encouraging list of self-help techniques and remedies with a track record of success is now available to MS patients.

Physically, self-help approaches work in three basic ways:

- by promoting a healthy immune system
- by stimulating the regeneration of healthy tissue
- by helping keep the blood–brain barrier intact

The interesting thing about the majority of self-help techiques is that the same things that help physical problems often also help psychological ones. So diet and lifestyle changes, for example, may not only stimulate regeneration of tissue but also make you feel mentally and emotionally stronger.

Better still, research is showing more and more that changes to our mental and emotional state can often have a powerful effect on our physical state as well. In other words, the mind and emotions can affect the body.

Self-help techniques effective for MS on both a physical and psychological level can be summarized as:

- modifing diet and improving nutrition (including cutting out food allergens)
- improving breathing
- taking regular exercise
- maintaining a positive outlook
- keeping your brain active and alert
- avoiding fatigue and controlling stress levels
- caring for your emotional and mental welfare

*Note* Because this book concentrates on positive treatment that can help keep MS at bay there is little information about practical aids for the very disabled such as how to acquire and use wheelchairs and incontinence pads. A wealth of information on help in these areas is already freely available in most countries from doctors, other books and the national charities listed in Appendix A.

## Diet and nutrition

Changing your diet and improving your nutritional intake are two of the most important ways to help yourself. Researchers have known for some time that fats play a major role in MS and so doing something about your fat intake is one of the most significant steps you can take. As Judy Graham says, 'shifting from a high saturated fat to a high *polyunsaturated* fat diet is probably the most important component of the self-help programme' in MS.

This is not only because saturated fats (such as animal fat) are believed to let toxins in the blood seep through into the brain but also because levels of the good essential fatty acids (EFAs) are abnormal in people with MS, and EFAs are only found in polyunsaturated fats (PUFAs). PUFAs play a vital role in the repair and maintenance of nerves and nerve tissue as well as blood health and brain activity.

Essential fatty acids come in two types. One type, known as omega-3 fatty acids, is found in sunflower and safflower seeds. It can also be taken as a food supplements – the best known being evening primrose oil. The other type is omega-6 fatty acids and you get it from oily fish such as herrings, mackerel and tuna as well as in dark green leafy vegetables. It, too, can be taken as a supplement, usually as fish or marine oils.

A range of other nutrients – vitamins, minerals and amino acids – known to be important in helping the body handle MS can also be taken as food supplements as well as part of a healthy diet.

Food supplements are nutrients concentrated and put into capsules or tablets (though some, such as vitamin C, are also popular in powder form) and taken as a supplement to a normal diet. The main nutrients helpful in MS (for repairing nerve tissue and protecting and boosting the immune system) are listed below.

### Vitamins

- *Vitamin A* (taken preferably as *beta-carotene*) An important antioxidant, beta-carotene is found in all green and yellow fruit and vegetables, particularly apricots, alfalfa, beetroot and carrots.
- *The B vitamins* All B vitamins are important in protecting the body against disease and infection as well as being helpful in repairing tissue and bolstering against the effects of stress. B3 (niacin) and B6 (pyridoxine) are also important in helping EFAs work properly. They are best taken as a 'complex' (the whole range together) but natural food sources are brewer's yeast, whole grains and meats such as liver and kidney.
- *Vitamin C* (ascorbic acid) Vitamin C stimulates the immune system to make *interferon*, a natural anti-viral agent. It is also antibiotic and antibacterial and helps EFAs to be processed properly in the body. Most fruit

and vegetables are sources (they must be fresh and raw) but especially citrus fruits, blackcurrants, rose-hips and peppers.

- *Vitamin D* This is found naturally in fish liver oils and eggs. The action of the sun on the skin also produces vitamin D in the body.
- *Vitamin E* The strongest of the antioxidants and often added in manufacturing to prevent oils like evening primrose oil and fish oils supplements 'oxidizing' or going rancid. Rancid matter in food produces damaging 'free radicals', unstable molecules described as the most potent toxin in the body and a powerful system of destruction.

## Minerals

- *Copper* This promotes energy by supporting the production of prostaglandins (see 'The Doctor's story', page 38) and helping the body use vitamin C and iron. Food sources are beans, peas, whole wheat, prunes, liver, seafood and green leafy vegetables.
- *Magnesium* Vital in the digestion of EFAs and in helping transmit nerve impulses to muscles. Some studies have shown people with MS are low in magnesium and others that magnesium supplements get rid of foot cramps, muscle spasms, involuntary twitching and inability to control the bladder. Food sources are almonds and sunflower and sesame seeds.
- *Manganese* One of the main supporters of the nervous system and active in combating auto-immune disease. Lack of manganese can produce disturbed balance (*ataxia*), fatigue, depression and allergies. Natural food sources are tropical fruit, nuts, cereals, egg yolk, and spices such as cloves, cardamom, ginger, turmeric and black pepper.
- *Molybdenum* A trace element normally low in people with MS. It is used by the body in the processing of

carbohydrates and fats and effective against mercury. Food sources are dark green leafy vegetables, whole grains and legumes (peas and beans).

- *Selenium* Another strong antioxidant and protector of cells from damage that works best with vitamins A, C and E. It particularly boosts the effectiveness of white blood cells to fight disease. Many people with MS are low in selenium. One of the best food sources is shellfish. Others are tuna, bran, onions, tomatoes and broccoli.
- *Vanadium* Needed to keep blood healthy. MS patients have been shown to be low in this trace element. Good food sources are parsley, radishes, lettuce, strawberries, sardines, cucumber and apples.
- *Zinc* Known as 'the immunity mineral', the mineral equivalent of vitamin C. The most widely-used mineral in the formation of enzymes, zinc has also a leading role in making sure vitamins, particularly the B vitamins, work properly and is essential for the production of prostaglandins from EFAs. Natural food sources are oysters, liver, eggs, fish, pumpkin seeds, beans, pulses, whole grains and brewer's yeast.

*Other supplements for MS*
Other food supplements said to be helpful in treating MS are:

- 'free form' *amino acids*, particularly methionine, taurine, cysteine/cystine, phenylalanine and tryptophan (amino acids are the basic protein 'building blocks' of life)
- *lecithin*, a polyunsaturated fat and a principal component of the brain (one of the best natural sources is eggs)
- *acidophilus* or *bifidophilus*, natural bacteria that promote a healthy gut, known generally as *probiotics* (a good food source is *live* yoghurt)

**Food supplements helpful for MS**

|  | Suggested dose |
|---|---|
| *Essential fatty acids* | |
| Evening primrose oil | 3x500mg three times daily |
| Fish oil | 1x1,000mg daily |
| *Vitamins* | |
| Vitamin C | 1x1g three times daily |
| Vitamin E | 1x1,000iu three times daily |
| B-complex | 1x25mg three times daily |
| Vitamin B6 | 1 or 2x50mg daily |
| Vitamin B12 | 1x1mg injection weekly |
| *Minerals* | |
| Magnesium | 1x200mg twice daily |
| Manganese | 1x10mg twice daily |
| Molybdenum | trace amounts |
| Selenium | 1x50mcg twice daily |
| Zinc | 1x15mg twice daily |
| *Others* | |
| Lecithin | 2x200mg three times daily |
| Amino acids | Half teaspoon twice daily |
| Acidophilus | 3x500mg daily |

*Note* It is possible to treat yourself using the above list but not advisable, mainly because of the high cost of doing so. It is best to consult a qualified nutritional therapist or naturopath who can tailor a programme to your specific needs. Injections can only be done by a doctor.

## Tips for healthy eating and drinking

- As far as possible buy organic and eat raw. Good, clean, fresh, organic, raw fruit and vegetables are the best foods to fight any disease.

- Eat sprouting seeds, the very simplest raw food. A small packet of organic *alfalfa* seeds, for example, would give you the equivalent of a bowl of raw vegetables every day for a week. Soak the seeds in water, rinse daily and eat when they start to sprout. Other good natural multi-nutrient foods are freshwater algae such as *chlorella* and *spirulina*. Widely popular in the Far East, they are usually sold in the West as dried powder.
- Give your body sustainable energy by eating slow-releasing carbohydrates such as whole grains, pulses, vegetables and fruit rather than sugar.
- Drink plenty of clean, filtered water (up to 2 litres/3½ pints a day if you can), diluted fruit juice or herb teas rather than tea, coffee or alcoholic drinks.
- Go to the toilet regularly. A good portion of raw foods each day will not only give you plenty of nutrients but enough fibre to keep your bowels healthy and ensure that waste matter is expelled quickly and efficiently as it should be.
- Wash all fruit and vegetables thoroughly before eating. Washing and then soaking them in a dilute solution of apple cider vinegar helps to take a lot of the contamination out of modern 'farmed foods'.
- Avoid sugary and saturated fatty foods. The most important foods to avoid in MS are:
  - fatty meat and all animal fats (including the skin of poultry, lard, dripping)
  - dairy products (*all* milk, including skimmed, semi-skimmed and low fat milk, butter, margarine, cheese and cream) and margarine, mayonnaise and salad cream
  - foods high in added sugar (cakes, biscuits/cookies, sweets/candies, pastries)

## The doctor's story

*Welsh doctor Bob Lawrence, 53, has successfully treated his own MS with a special dietary programme he is now making available to others.*

Bob Lawrence suspected he had MS when he was 35, ten years before he was officially diagnosed in 1986. As a doctor he knew conventional medicine had little to offer him except steroids and immunosuppressant drugs.

'Drugs such as steroids used in the treatment of MS are not only ineffective in halting the progress of the disease but can hasten further deterioration by suppressing adrenal function and further disrupting the immune system,' he says.

The result was he decided to try and work out his own treatment based on research into *prostaglandins*, a vital type of essential fatty acid that plays a key role in the healthy working of the immune system.

Since his forced retirement in 1986 he has developed a programme based on a combination of diet and food supplements that he says has helped to stabilize his condition and, above all, given him more energy.

'Fatigue is one of the biggest problems for people with MS but I think I've managed to discover a combination that can overcome that,' he says. 'It has certainly worked for me.

'I've been stable for seven years now – though I've also been using hyperbaric oxygen (see *page 88*). It helped but I've now stopped it because it's increased my angina.'

Dr Lawrence finally decided his results were good enough to develop for the benefit of other people and in 1991 he set up a company to manufacture and distribute his method, which he calls the 'Zenwa Diet'.

This is based largely on the elimination of all saturated fat (such as red meat), 'significant' allergy foods (such as gluten, eggs, dairy products, caffeine and additives), strong curries and spices, and 'large' quantities of refined sugar – and supplementing with essential fatty acids (oil from evening primrose, borage seed, sunflower, fish-liver and flaxseed), the minerals zinc, copper, selenium and magnesium, and the vitamins B-complex, A, C and E.

'The neurologist who advised me said that despite the work of Professor Swank in America diet was of no possible benefit for MS – but I now know he was wrong.'

You can find out more about his work from Dietary Research Ltd, University Innovation Centre, Singleton Park, Swansea, West Glamorgan SA2 8PP, Wales, UK (tel 01792 295562, fax 01792 295613).

## Allergies

Food and drink supply the body with a lot of the energy it needs to function but they can cause problems when they contain toxic chemicals such as artificial colouring, preservatives, additives, pesticides or growth enhancers (added during processing), or where there is something wrong with the body they enter.

This can lead to what is known as an 'allergic reaction' and the person is then said to suffer from 'food allergies'. Some specialists claim MS sufferers typically have allergies to any number of foods but especially tea, milk, potatoes, gluten (wheat), sugar, yeast and citrus fruits.

Judy Graham reported that eliminating tea, coffee, sugar, milk and yeast from her diet produced an almost overnight transformation: 'It was like a sort of fog lifting, and had a dramatic effect on banishing fatigue.'

Sensitivities and intolerances (or allergies) to foods can be tested in a variety of ways. The best self-help method is by following what is called an 'exclusion' or 'elimination diet'. By excluding or eliminating various foods from your diet one after the other you isolate the ones that make you react or feel bad.

This is a laborious process of trial-and-error and needs to be done with great care to be accurate. Many people find it better to see a recommended therapist who specializes in testing for allergies scientifically (see *Chapter 7*).

## Improving breathing

Learning to breathe properly is an easy self-help method that can help any problem but is particularly useful in MS.

Correct breathing is breathing with the abdomen, or stomach, not the chest (see *figure 6*). Babies and young children do this naturally and what it does is push the *diaphragm*, the domed-shaped sheet of muscle which separates the stomach and the bottom of the lungs, upwards. This in turn pushes out air in the very bottom of the lungs and stops stale air collecting there.

Chest or *thoracic* breathing, as it is correctly known, tends to mean that only air in the top half of the lungs is expelled.

The best way to change the air in your lungs is to exercise. You can take in as much as 3 litres (5 pints) of air with each breath when you exercise, thus clearing the whole of your lungs in just two or three breaths.

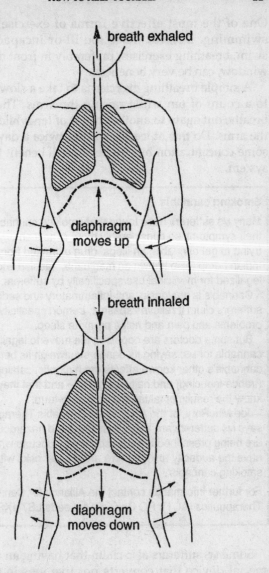

**Fig. 6 Breathing correctly**

One of the most effective forms of exercise for MS is swimming. But, for those too ill or incapacitated to swim, breathing exercises, preferably in front of an open window, can be very beneficial.

A simple breathing exercise is to take a slow breath in to a count of ten while raising the arms. Then slowly breathe out again to another count of ten while lowering the arms. Do this at least ten times twice a day. It needs some concentration but the result will benefit the whole system.

---

### Smoking cannabis

Many MS sufferers have found that smoking cannabis helps their symptoms so considerably there is now an organization trying to get cannabis, an illegal drug extracted from the herb Indian hemp (also known as marijuana, hashish and ganja), legalized for medicinal use specifically by sufferers.

Cannabis is analgesic, anti-inflammatory and sedative and sufferers claim it relieves spasms, tremor, spasticity, bladder problems and pain and helps promote sleep.

But some doctors are opposing the move to legalize cannabis for MS, saying its dangers outweigh its benefits – cannabis's other known effects are hypnotic, cataleptic (trance-inducing) and hallucinogenic – and that they do not know the results of taking the drug long-term.

Joe MacRory, of the Alliance for Cannabis Therapeutics, says MS sufferers are angry that 'toxic and hazardous drugs are being prescribed in every country by doctors who then have the audacity to infer there are greater risks with smoking cannabis'.

For further information contact the Alliance for Cannabis Therapeutics (ACT), PO Box CR14, Leeds LS7 4XF, UK.

---

Some MS sufferers also claim that having an *ionizer* – a special device that converts positive ions in the air to healthy negative ions – in the room helps.

Good posture also encourages proper breathing. Sitting or standing with your shoulders hunched reduces lung capacity greatly. Sitting or standing straight with shoulders back expands the lungs. Learning to hold the body and expand the lungs naturally gives extra space to all internal organs.

One of the best ways to learn how to improve the posture is the Alexander Technique (see *Chapter 7*).

## Andrew's story

*Former businessman Andrew found that nothing worked so well for his MS as regular cold baths.*

Andrew, 40, from Enfield, south-east England, was not diagnosed officially as suffering from MS until 1994 – 15 years after first showing symptoms.

Despite suffering complete and unremitting numbness over his entire body since the age of 24, starting with an icy numbness in his fingertips that spread slowly, no one, including some of Britain's top MS doctors, would confirm MS, says Andrew.

After eight years of this he finally paid for a scan himself – costing £475 (US $713) – because his doctors refused to let him have it on the state. ('They said it would be a waste of money.') The scan confirmed advanced MS in his brain.

Andrew was not put off by the result. He had already suspected he had MS and had started fighting back. 'I have tried and will try anything so long as it is not drugs,' he says. 'Specialists have tried me on various drugs like steroids and muscle relaxants and they haven't made the slightest difference.'

So far he has tried homoeopathy, acupuncture, Chinese herbs, hypnotherapy, massage, electro-magnetic therapy and cold bath therapy.

He says the herbs helped a little and the massage a lot – but the benefits did not last. The thing that worked best was regular cold baths.

'A friend told me about it in the spring of 1994 and so every day I sat in cold water for about half an hour. It was difficult at first but I soon got used to it.

'After about a month I felt and looked so much better I increased to two baths a day. From lasting for about two hours afterwards the effect then lasted for five or six hours. During that time I felt 99 per cent normal.'

But summer ended the benefit. 'During the summer I couldn't get the water cold enough, no matter how early I got up or how long I ran it. I found it didn't work if the temperature was above 16°C [61°F].'

The benefits didn't last after he stopped the baths but Andrew still says he would recommend the therapy to anyone: 'It really worked for me. It was brilliant.'

*Caution* Cold baths are a recognized and well-documented therapy of benefit to the immune system but some people with MS might be made worse by them. Extremely cold baths are also not recommended for anyone with a heart problem without a medical checkup first.

## Taking regular exercise

As explained in *chapter 2* an important part in treating MS is knowing that there is nothing wrong with the muscles. The muscles of people with MS are healthy. But they become unhealthy if they are not used, contracting into fixed positions or wasting away. So it is extremely important in MS that muscles are kept working – and that means exercising them.

Regular exercise can make the difference between being able to stand or walk and becoming wheelchair-bound. Almost any exercise is better than none but the most beneficial for MS are the following:

- *Swimming* This can have therapeutic as well as exercise benefits so long as the water isn't too hot. Therapeutically-speaking water treatment is known as hydrotherapy (see *box 'Andrew's story'* and *Chapter 7*).
- *Dancing* People can get away with doing almost anything on the dance floor these days so no one is going to notice if you are not as coordinated as some others!
- *Using toning and exercise machines* or a *mini-trampoline* (sometimes called a 'rebounder').

Two of the most effective ways of exercising are yoga and exercises developed just for people with MS. Both have been shown to be highly beneficial.

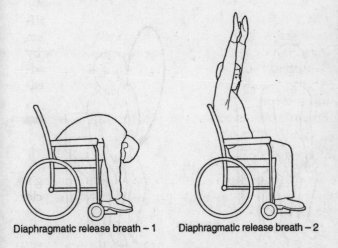

Diaphragmatic release breath – 1    Diaphragmatic release breath – 2

**Fig. 7  Yoga breathing exercise for the wheelchair-bound**

## Yoga

Work by the Yoga for Health Foundation in Britain has found yoga can keep people with MS mobile and active as well as mentally and emotionally fit – even those confined to a wheelchair (see *figure 7*). There is more about yoga in *Chapters 7* and *8*.

## Exercises for MS

British physical therapist and MS sufferer Susie Cornell has pioneered an entire programme of exercises for people with MS after she became dissatisfied with the standard approach of most physiotherapists to MS. Her motto – fully approved of by more forward-looking physiotherapists – is 'use it or lose it'.

An example of a simple exercise for coordination is shown in *figure 8*. Another is her simple tip to keep hands and arms strong: carry around a tennis ball or soft sponge-ball with you and squeeze it as often as possible throughout the day (see also *'Susie's story', pages 77–8*).

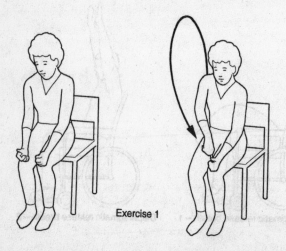

Exercise 1

**Fig. 8 Coordination exercises for MS**

*Exercise 1*

Sit properly on a chair with both feet on the ground and place your clenched fists on your knees with the thumbs pointing up. Keeping your arm straight and your thumb sticking up, swing your right arm backwards as if doing the 'front crawl' stroke in swimming and, to a count of five, bring it down and across your body to join the thumb on your left knee. Return to your right knee by reversing the movement, still to a count of five. Do this using each finger in turn and then switch to do the same with your left thumb and fingers to your right knee.

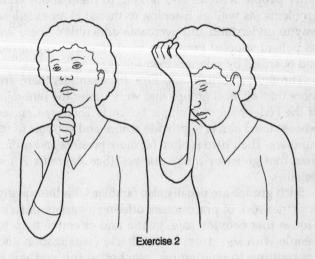

Exercise 2

*Exercise 2*

Still sitting with your fists clenched on your knees and your thumbs up, move your right thumb to touch the point of your chin and back down again. Then your nose and back down again. Then place the inside of your wrist on to your forehead and bring it back. Repeat both movements using your left thumb and then each finger of both hands in turn.

## Keeping a healthy mental and emotional outlook

Scientists now know that severe stress and strain can cause blood toxins to break through into the brain – where they do not belong – and in MS this has been shown to play a crucial part in the development of the disease. In addition, feeling depressed and helpless affects the way your body handles essential fatty acids.

Nurture and care for yourself, and if you need more help than your family and friends can give you, try your family doctor. If he or she can't or won't help, meeting other people with MS and talking to them about your problems (as well as listening to theirs) is an excellent way to understand and overcome difficulties. There are MS patient support groups in most countries organized and operated by sufferers themselves.

Throughout Britain and Eire, for example, there are more than 60 local groups that work under the umbrella of the Federation of Multiple Sclerosis Therapy Centres whose stated aim is to provide advice and support to MS sufferers. Their help is often far more positive and useful than that given by many doctors. (See *Appendix A* for details.)

Such groups are usually also familiar with the equally wide network of practitioners offering a variety of techniques that provide safe, gentle and effective help to people with MS – from biofeedback, visualization and counselling to meditation, psychotherapy and yoga. These are described in more detail in *Chapter 8*.

First, however, we will look at the sort of conventional treatment you might receive for MS.

# CHAPTER 5

# Conventional treatments and procedures

*What your doctor is likely to say and do*

Despite recent advances, MS is still one of those conditions doctors class as chronic (long-term) for which there is no known cause, cure or treatment. As most of the stories in this book make clear, the majority of doctors feel they can do little.

In both diagnosis and treatment MS remains a disease doctors generally are uneasy about and handle badly.

The main problem for doctors is that MS is not the only disease of the central nervous system. Conditions as relatively temporary and harmless as *neuralgia* (pain from an irritated or damaged nerve), *neuritis* (inflammation of a nerve), *sciatica* (irritation of the sciatic nerve), *slipped disc* and spine problems can all cause symptoms of tingling and numbness.

Serious diseases of the nervous system and muscles other than MS include *Parkinson's disease*, *Guillain-Barré syndrome*, *Huntingdon's chorea* and *motor neurone disease*.

Symptoms such as severe headache and sensitivity to bright light are more likely to be the result of something else entirely such as *migraine*.

## The diagnosis

One of the biggest problems with MS is the lack of early diagnosis. Most doctors find it hard to diagnose MS early with any confidence. They will usually wait for at least three different attacks or 'episodes' to occur, often over some years, before confirming a diagnosis. But the very serious problem with this 'delayed diagnosis' approach is that it can allow a manageable condition to become an unmanageable one.

Most doctors these days will start to suspect MS if your first symptom, or even one of your symptoms, is blurred, dimmed or double vision. The cause is probably inflammation of the optic nerve carrying signals from the eye to the brain, a condition known medically as *optic neuritis*.

Impaired eyesight is the single most important indicator of MS. Up to 40 per cent of all MS starts this way and up to 75 per cent of MS patients suffer from it at some stage (though impaired vision can, of course, be caused by many other things as well and so is not a gaurantee you have MS).

But if your symptoms are tingling or numbness in the hands or feet, another common first sign, it is much less certain you have MS. Tension, anxiety and hyperventilation (over-breathing) are the most likely causes and may be corrected simply enough with any of the relaxation therapies described in this book.

Apart from taking a medical history and doing a few basic tests such as testing coordination and reflexes with a hammer (the 'knee jerk' test) and pin, most family doctors consider themselves ill-equipped to make a diagnosis of MS and so will almost certainly refer you as soon as possible to a specialist in nerves, known as a *neurologist*. This would be at your nearest specialist centre – usually a main hospital, where you will receive a range of tests.

## Electrophysiological tests

One of the first tests to be done is usually what doctors call the *visual, auditory and somatosensory evoked potentials test*. This uses electrodes placed on the head to send small electrical impulses to different parts of the brain to measure the time between the brain being stimulated and the body responding. The 'message' takes longer to get through in people with MS – a factor known medically as the *electrophysiological deficit*.

This test is not confirmation of MS but suggests it as a possibility. Someone with suspected MS will then normally go for more analytical laboratory tests as below.

## Lumbar puncture

A lumbar puncture is the oldest procedure for diagnosing MS, and still the standard in many areas. It involves a needle being inserted under local anaesthetic into the spine (in the small of the back) and syphoning off for analysis some of the fluid around the spinal cord (the *cerebro-spinal fluid*). MS may be confirmed if there are traces of myelin sheath in the fluid.

The procedure is highly invasive, quite dangerous and not, unfortunately, fool-proof. Short- and long-term after-effects can be very unpleasant. Some people report a headache so severe they are unable to lift their head from the pillow for days afterwards, for example. Worst of all, its results are not conclusive proof of MS.

## Myelogram

A myelogram is an x-ray of the spinal cord after the injection of a dye into the spine that the x-ray can track. This, also, is not confirmation of MS but it is used to try and identify any blockages in the nerves and so eliminate other possible causes of the symptoms the person is experiencing.

## Magnetic resonance imager

A magnetic resonance imager (MRI) is the latest in high-tech diagnostic equipment. It is a 'whole body' scanner linked to a computer that makes use of magnetic force fields, 50,000 times stronger than that of the Earth, to build up a detailed and accurate 'picture' of the body. It is a slow and, for some, uncomfortable process but its accuracy is such that specialists say they can detect around 95 per cent of any damage to myelin sheath (neither x-rays nor CT – 'Cat' – scans are of any use in the diagnosis of MS this way).

MRI is proving invaluable in detecting damage in those areas of the body such as the brain and spinal cord where methods of investigation such as surgery are difficult and dangerous. Unfortunately the cost of the equipment is so high it is still far from being a standard procedure in most countries. Also, its long-term effects are uncertain.

## Other tests available

Among more recent, and therefore less common, tests are two blood tests that promise to become much more widely available as their value is proven.

## Immunoglobulin estimations

Immunoglobulins (written Ig for short) are particular substances in white blood cells called 'antibodies'. As part of the body's immune system, their job is to recognize, seek out and help destroy 'antigens' – that is, organisms coming into the body that are bad for the body such as infections.

There are five types of immunoglobulins, identified with the letters of the alphabet. Immunoglobulin G (IgG) accounts for 70 per cent of antibodies and is responsible for long-term immunity. Researchers have found that more than half of those with MS have an abnormal proportion of IgG in their blood. The IgG estimations test measures the proportions of the different immunoglobulins and is likely to become rapidly more in use in MS diagnosis as the test is refined.

*Electrophoretic mobility test*

People with MS seem to have an abnormal essential fatty acids profile in their blood cells, particularly of the types known as *linoleic acid* and *arachidonic acid*. The electrophoretic mobility test picks up these abnormalities.

## The treatment

On the basis of some or all of the tests a diagnosis will be made and treatment, if any, start. The results may be made known to you but sometimes, for the reasons explained, doctors say they either aren't sure or lie about the outcome.

However the treatment you get is the clearest indication you have of whether your doctor thinks you have MS.

The conventional treatment for MS is normally prescription drugs. These are for 'dampening down' inflammation during attacks, dealing with any urinary problems and relieving the pain of spastic muscles. Doctors may also prescribe antidepressants and, less commonly, refer patients for physiotherapy and counselling.

Remember, conventional treatment contains nothing like the range of therapies available in non-conventional medicine and, even though those that are available are potent and improving all the time, *none is a cure*. Also, most conventional treatment, unlike natural medicine, tends to concentrate on treating surface symptoms rather than root causes.

## Drugs

The standard drug treatments for MS for many years are the following:

- steroids
- antispasmodics and anticholinergics
- muscle relaxants
- antidepressants
- pain-killers

### Steroids

Steroids are powerful anti-inflammatory drugs and are usually given during an attack of MS by daily direct injection into the veins (known as an *intravenous infusion*) over a period of three to five days, followed by a steroid pill for ten days. Treatment has proved effective in reducing symptoms of MS and getting people back on their feet, but it is not a cure.

The main steroids used in MS are:

- *adrenocorticotrophic hormone* (ACTH)
- *methylprednisolone*

The trouble with steroids is that they go for short-term gain at long-term expense. In MS they may reduce symptoms, and so are useful in the management of attacks, but they weaken the immune system.

Immediate side-effects include raised blood pressure, raised blood sugar and other chemical imbalances sometimes leading to a feeling of being 'spaced out'.

Long-term effects of continuous steroid use include swelling ('moon face'), weight gain, unwanted hair, delayed wound-healing, eye problems such as *glaucoma* and *cataracts*, impotence, ulcers, kidney stones, diabetes and *osteoporosis*, the thinning and weakening of bones.

## Barbara's story

*Former teacher Barbara, 37, has been told by her doctors they can do nothing for her except give her drugs and occasional physiotherapy.*

Barbara experienced her first symptoms of MS in 1988 – three weeks after the birth of her first child. Her family doctor thought she might be suffering from post-natal depression – but he was unsure enough to send her for tests.

The tests – Barbara describes them as a 'frightening experience' – confirmed MS but Barbara was not told. She was not formally told until two years later, when her sight suddenly went (it returned later).

Against her consultant's advice, who felt her pregnancy had triggered her MS, she became pregnant again with her second son in 1991 but did not suffer a recurrence of the earlier collapse.

Barbara now has a twice-yearly course of intravenous steroid injections over a five-day period, takes pain-killers constantly and antidepressants for occasional bouts of depression.

'My doctor sends me for physiotherapy when I need it and I go to the gym for regular work-outs,' says Barbara. 'I believe if I don't use parts of my body as I'm meant to I'll lose them.'

Even though Barbara hates the steroids – 'they make you feel totally spaced out and put on weight' – and did stop taking them for a while she says her consultant insists she continue with them.

'I argue with him but not too much. I feel if I did stop them he wouldn't see me any more.'

At the end of 1994 her speech went completely and so she agreed to yet another course. She feels they helped her recovery, even though she knows they are

not a cure. She has thought, she says, of trying other
methods said to be effective 'but not too much'.

Neither her family doctor nor her consultant have
suggested she try anything else.

Today she considers herself relatively stable, though
her left leg has never recovered from her first attack
and she lives in fear of not recovering from subse-
quent relapses.

## Antispasmodics and anticholinergics

Antispasmodics treat the sense of bladder 'urgency' and
incontinence often suffered by people with MS by interfering with the parasympathetic nervous system that
controls the action of the bladder. Examples of those
used in MS are *oxybutynin* (brand names Cystrin – UK
only – and Ditropan) and *flavoxate* (brand name Urispas).

Anticholinergics are used to relieve muscle ache and
stiffness. A common example is the antiviral drug
*amantadine*, also used to treat severe flu infection.

Antispasmodics and anticholinergics can cause
headache, nausea, fatigue, dry mouth, blurred vision
and diarrhoea. Other side-effects are flushing,
constipation and irregular heartbeat.

## Muscle relaxants

Benzodiazepines relax muscles by interfering with nerve
signals. One of the best-known examples is *diazepam*
(brand names Valium and Diazepam) but the versions
most commonly used in MS are *baclofen* (Lioresal) which
acts at the spinal level and *dantrolene* (Dantrium).
Benzodiazepines are addictive and side-effects include
drowsiness, slow reactions and varicose veins. *Baclofen*
can cause nausea, reduced alertness, low blood pressure,
muscle ache, lowered heart and breathing rate, visual
disturbances and rash. Dantrolene can cause liver failure.

*Antidepressants*

Antidepressants are used to treat the depression that often goes with MS by interfering with the chemistry of the brain. It is not an attempt to remove or overcome the depression so much as to suppress it.

Antidepressants (also known as *psychoactive* drugs) commonly used in MS are of two main types:

- *tricyclics*, or TCAD: common examples are *lofepramine* (brand name Gamanil), *dothiepin* (Prothiaden), *amitriptyline* (Trytizol)
- *selective serotonin reuptake inhibitors*, or SSRIs: the best-known example is *fluoxetine* (brand name Prozac)

As with any strong drug, antidepressants have numerous side-effects, many extremely serious. With tricyclic drugs they include confusion, memory problems, delirium, disorientation, dry mouth, fatigue, blurred vision, sexual dysfunction, palpitations, drowsiness, rapid heartbeat, excessive sweating and disturbed concentration.

Common side-effects of SSRIs include anxiety, insomnia, nausea, tremors, vomiting, diarrhoea and upset stomach, weight and appetite changes, convulsions, dizziness, headaches, drowsiness, fever, rash, and allergic reactions.

Despite these side-effects most doctors tend to believe that depression is better treated with drugs than non-drug therapy – though a change may be under way (see *Counselling*, page 61).

*Pain-killers*

Pain-killers, known as 'analgesics' to doctors, include anything from *aspirin* and *paracetamol* for mild to moderate pain to a variety of opium-based drugs such as *buprenorphine* (UK brand name Temgesic and US brand name Buprenex) for severe pain. Analgesics in general depress the central nervous system and some are addictive but, again, in cases of severe pain may be unavoidable and essential.

### Latest developments in drug treatments

Recently new drugs have been developed that promise to revolutionize the treatment of MS – though specialists are stressing they are unlikely to replace the use of steroids as a 'first aid' treatment for relapse, and they are not a cure.

### Immunosuppressants

Developed for use mainly in transplant operations to prevent organ rejection, doctors now consider they could be useful in the treatment of some auto-immune diseases including MS. The best known drug in this range is *cyclosporin* (brand name Sandimmun). Other examples are *methotrexate* (Maxtrex) and *mitozantrone* (Novantrone).

Immunosuppressants work by suppressing the immune system, thus reducing the ability of the body to fight infection. This frequently allows other infections such as the yeast infection *candidiasis* to develop that might not otherwise occur. Medical opinion is divided about whether immunosuppressants have any value in MS but research into their use for MS is continuing.

### Immunomodulators

These drugs are so named because they seem to work by modulating or regulating the immune system – that is, adjusting any under- or over-reaction – so it works more efficiently. Trials of two, *beta-interferon* and *copolymer-1*, had produced such good results by the end of 1994 that they are likely to be licensed for limited general use. Indeed beta-interferon, the most promising of the two, already has been licensed in America.

*Beta-interferon* is a complex synthetic protein that partly mimics natural interferon, an antiviral agent made naturally by the body's immune system.

Its precise action is not fully understood yet but it seems to improve the function of the immune system by 'fine-tuning' it in some way as well as reducing the increase of harmful cells and acting as an antiviral agent.

Two large clinical trials announced in 1993–4 showed that beta-interferon was successful in reducing the severity of attacks by half and lessening the frequency of attacks by a third, thus 'significantly' delaying deterioration. MRI scans showed that myelin sheath damage was reduced by just over half in people on the drug for two years – leading to a possible delay in the onset of disability.

Medical opinion in 1995 was that beta-interferon was likely to be most effective for people with relapsing–remitting MS in the early stages. It still needs to be tested for chronic progressive MS.

---

**The latest on beta-interferon**

Two types of beta-interferon are currently available. Each has a different composition and is produced in a different way. Interferon beta 1a, produced in the UK with the trade name *Rebif*, is expected to be launched on general prescription before 1997 at the end of extensive trials still going on. But it is already available privately to people in the UK prepared to pay up to £30,000 (US $45,000) a year for the treatment.

Interferon beta 1b is produced in the USA under the trade name *Betaseron* and has been in use by MS patients in America since October 1993. It is expected to be launched in Europe in 1996 as *Beneseron*.

---

*Copolymer-1* was first announced in October 1994 at a joint meeting of American and British neurologists. It resembles a part of the tissue in myelin sheath and, like beta-interferon, was developed for MS on the basis of laboratory experiments with cell technology.

How it works is also still something of a mystery but it is believed to fool the immune system into working correctly by desensitizing or 'shutting down' faulty cells in myelin.

*Caution* Despite the promise of immunomodulators for MS they are still experimental and leading experts in Britain and elsewhere are officially urging caution while more trials are carried out and more evidence collected.

They point out that the existing US licence is limited to use only in early relapsing–remitting MS and is conditional on clinical benefits being confirmed over a long period.

Professor Ian McDonald, senior physician at the National Hospital of Neurology and Neurosurgery in London and a leading expert on MS, said early in 1995 he believes immunomodulators are likely to have a wider role in the management of MS but cautioned against expectations being too high.

He said he believes the drugs may prove effective in the early stages of the disease for those who are only slightly to moderately affected but not necessarily in the long term. He does not believe they are a substitute for steroids to manage relapses.

Immediate side-effects of beta-interferon reported so far include flu-like symptoms and some irritation where the drug is injected (patients are taught how to inject themselves in the same way diabetics use insulin). It also increases depression in some people.

### Physiotherapy and exercise

Conventional medicine encourages exercise as a way to maintain mobility generally but does not automatically refer someone with MS for physiotherapy (physical therapy). A physiotherapist is specially trained to exercise muscles to improve mobility. But physiotherapy is regarded by many MS sufferers as neither as thorough nor as helpful as a dedicated exercise routine (see *Chapter 7*).

**'Oral tolerization' – a new hope?**

Doctors in America who see MS as a purely auto-immune disease are developing a 'gentle' new treatment based on some of the ideas in traditional Chinese medicine which they are calling 'oral tolerization'.

Patients are basically given minute amounts of myelin protein to eat. Eating rather than injecting the protein is important. The body is immediately suspicious of anything injected into the body but it rarely turns against food. The theory is that if the protein is taken in through the gut the body will learn to tolerate what it is that is faulty in myelin tissue and accept it instead of turning against it.

MS specialist Dr Howard Weiner, an immunologist at the Harvard Medical School in Boston, has called oral tolerization 'a form of vaccination via the gut'. He says it works by shutting down only the part of the body that has been causing the trouble rather than affecting the immune system as a whole like steroids and other drugs.

He claims it is a safe and simple treatment that has already shown success in preliminary trials. Patients have been able to stop or cut back on standard drugs. A fullscale trial of more than 400 people with MS in the USA and Canada began in spring 1995. Doctors hope it will prove the value of the treatment but results will not be known for some time.

## Counselling

In recent years a growing number of doctors have woken up to the benefits of counselling over antidepressant drugs. A study in the *British Medical Journal* in March 1995 showed that 'problem-solving' approaches gave better results than antidepressants for depression. Not only are more doctors prepared to offer counselling but trained professional counsellors are now a more common feature of many medical units.

An alternative to counselling, though rather less popular or common in a conventional medical setting (except in America), is psychotherapy (see *Chapter 8* ).

## Surgery for MS

Surgery is not a treatment traditionally thought of in connection with MS but a new technique being developed in America claims to be helping people with severe disability, particularly those with convulsive-type tremors, to recover some control of muscles.

The technique is *thalamotomy* and it involves directing electronic heat impulses by an electrode inserted into the brain to interrupt and block the electrical pathways sending the faulty signals. The electrode is guided by a computer linked to an MRI scanner.

The technique is being pioneered at Texas Southwestern Medical Center in Dallas and so far about a dozen sufferers have been helped, though doctors are stressing it is not a cure.

## The follow-up

In cases where MS causes a general deterioration to the stage of serious disability, doctors will call in occupational therapists to care for and advise a sufferer and give them reports. By this stage it may have become clear that remission is unlikely (though not impossible) and that the disease has progressed to a point of no return.

Doctors continue to monitor and have a responsibility for the patient and intervene where deterioration causes life-threatening complications or side-effects. Patients too disabled to travel are usually supervised by a district nurse. Social workers may also be involved to help with social and financial problems such as benefit payments.

# CHAPTER 6

# The natural therapies and MS

*Introducing the 'gentle alternatives'*

There is little that is new about most natural therapies. The majority of the treatments involved, from massage to the use of herbs and water, are probably as old as the art of healing itself. Some, such as Chinese medicine and *Ayurveda* (traditional Indian medicine), have a pedigree thousands of years old.

The rise of modern 'scientific' medicine in the last 200 years has resulted in many of these ancient practices being pushed into the background, and even suppressed. But in recent years that trend has been dramatically reversed. Natural therapies are becoming as popular and widespread as they ever were.

The return of traditional medicine (conventional medicine is *new* medicine, not traditional) has resulted in a host of new ideas entering the already wide 'menu' of therapies, from homoeopathy to the more recent reflexology and radionics, and the list increases almost daily. The variety of therapies available can be daunting, and certainly makes choice extremely hard for the majority of those not brought up in the 'natural' tradition.

The remainder of this book sets out to make that choice a lot clearer and easier.

## Why go to a natural therapist?

A natural health practitioner is, or should be, someone who understands not only you and your problem but is also familiar with the host of safe and gentle treatments that do not involve your being either filled with unpleasant drugs or operated on, and who is prepared to give you plenty of time to explore these options.

People often turn to a natural therapist as a last resort. They have tried the conventional route and it hasn't worked. For whatever reason – and it may be because their problem was not helped or, sadly, perhaps even made worse – their needs haven't been met.

Whatever the reasons why people go to practitioners of natural therapy they seem to get a high level of satisfaction when they do. In Britain, for example, where no therapist is legally required to train to practise non-medical therapy, surveys in recent years have consistently shown satisfaction levels between 60 and 80 per cent.

## What is natural therapy?

There is a quite a discussion (not to say argument, even among natural therapists themselves) about whether all natural therapies operate under one common idea or principle.

The British Medical Association, in a report it published in June 1993, said they did not – that the natural therapies were a mish-mash of different styles and techniques with nothing in common at all. But this is not true. The natural approaches more or less all understand, accept and operate under the following principles:

- The body has a natural ability to heal itself and remain stable (this is known medically as *homoeostatis*)
- The human being is not simply a physical machine, like a car, but a subtle and complex blend of body,

mind and emotions (or spirit or soul as some prefer to call it) and that all or any of these factors may cause or contribute to problems of health. In other words, that every individual is not a random collection of moving parts but a fully integrated 'whole'. The term 'holistic medicine' has been coined to describe treating the individual as a 'whole being' composed of body, mind and emotions.

- Environmental and social conditions are just as important as a person's physical and psychological makeup and may have just as big an impact on their health.

- Treating the root cause or causes of a problem is more important than treating the obvious immediate symptoms. Treating only symptoms may simply cover up the real underlying problem and make it worse, so that it reappears later as something much more serious.

- Each person is an entirely original individual and cannot be treated in exactly the same way as every other person.

- Healing is quicker and more effective if the person takes central responsibility for his or her own health and has an active involvement in the healing process (but a good therapist will also recognize when someone needs to 'let go' and place themselves in the hands of another).

- Good health is a state of emotional, mental, spiritual and physical 'balance'. Balance is fundamental to the basic notion of health in natural therapy. Ill-health, say its exponents, is the result of being in a state of imbalance, or 'dis-ease'. The Chinese express this as the principle of *yin* and *yang*.

- There is a natural healing 'force' in the universe (the Chinese call this *qi* or *chi* – pronounced 'chee' – the Japanese *ki*, Indians *prana*. In the West it used to be called by its Latin description *vis medicatrix naturae*, meaning 'natural healing force', shortened today to 'life force'). Anyone can 'tap into' or make use of this force and it is a natural health practitioner's skill to activate it in the patient or help the patient activate it in themselves.

It is natural therapists' belief in the Oriental ideas expressed particularly in the last two principles – and also often their use of those terms – that have caused so much controversy among so many doctors trained in the Western scientific method. It is frequently the single most important reason they reject so much of it.

In summary, natural therapists believe that the best approach is the one that is the softest and gentlest, that avoids dangerous and traumatic procedures, that treats the patient as a 'whole' individual, and in which the patient takes an active part in his or her own recovery and health maintenance.

## The sorts of natural therapy

- *Physical therapies* These work obviously and directly on the body in a very physical way, both outside and in. Examples are chiropractic, herbalism, osteopathy, nutritional therapy and massage.
- *Psychological therapies* These aim to benefit the mind and emotions. Examples are meditation, psychotherapy, hypnotherapy, counselling, relaxation therapy and biofeedback.
- *'Energy' therapies* These are often based on Eastern ideas of health and disease (or dis-ease) and work on the idea that illness is the result of an imbalance or interruption in the body's natural energy or 'life force' at a very fine or subtle level. Examples are acupuncture, homoeopathy, reflexology and shiatsu.

Categories like this are never quite satisfactory, though, and there are many therapies which fall into more than one of the above headings. That is, they have a 'multi-level' effect, benefiting both body and mind as well as, in some people's view, the soul or spirit of a person. A good example of this is yoga but others would be massage and meditation.

*Note* Because MS is such a complex disease, with many possible causes producing a wide variety of symptoms different in almost every individual, no therapy on its own is likely to offer 'the' magic cure. Most people who have been helped have had to find the right combination of self-help and therapies that worked for them.

---

### Judy's story

British author and broadcaster Judy Graham, 47, has successfully treated her chronic progressive MS with a variety of self-help approaches and natural therapies.

Judy was officially diagnosed as having MS when she was 27. Determined not to give in to the disease she fought back so successfully she today claims to be able to lead a near normal life, 'juggling career, child, partner and home.'

Natural therapies that helped Judy were acupuncture, osteopathy, homoeopathy, hydrotherapy, herbalism, applied kinesiology, massage, reflexology and electromagnetic therapy.

She has also tried hyperbaric oxygen therapy with success: 'I am living proof that you don't have to get worse once you have MS. It is possible to stablilize, and even improve.'

## Peter's story

*London marketing executive Peter, 38, has successfully fought MS by trying a wide range of natural therapies and maintaining a 'fighting spirit'.*

Peter did not develop symptoms of MS until he was 35. A series of tests, and finally a scan by magnetic resonance imager (MRI), revealed MS-like lesions on the nerves to his eyes.

The symptoms at that stage were so small, only slightly affecting his eyesight, he did not take the diagnosis seriously – until three months later when he had a severe attack that affected almost the whole of his right side, accompanied by a burning pain in the arm.

The effects lasted months and Peter ran the gamut of emotions, believing that from being a fit and active sportsman he would soon be in a wheelchair: 'At first I could do nothing but cry and ask, why me? I thought, that's it, I'd had it. I was devastated. I simply don't know how I coped.'

But then he made the crucial decision to fight back. Within an hour of being officially diagnosed he was back at work and, determined not to give in, threw himself into building up his business, working harder than ever.

He also decided that since nothing conventional medicine had to offer could help him he would look elsewhere, and so he turned to natural medicine.

'The doctors, and I paid for the best, said they could do nothing. They said they could offer me only steroids. I tried them and they didn't seem to do any good so I stopped after the first course.'

In the last three years – during which he has had

two further attacks lasting up to three months – he says he has tried a wide range of alternative therapies.

'Some helped and some didn't. I had all my mercury fillings replaced, but that made no difference – though I'm glad I had them done – I had intravenous hydrogen peroxide injections that also didn't seem to help, and I tried faith healing.

'The things I think helped and I still carry on with are homoeopathy, diet – I eat no red meat, dairy products or gluten – food supplements, kinesiology, a form of hi-tech reflexology known as Vacuflex, lymphatic massage, cranial osteopathy and acupuncture.

'If I hear of any others I'll try those too. I'll try anything that might work. I simply refuse to give in to this thing. The fact that allopathic medicine has got nothing to offer – nothing at all, it's a complete waste of time – means that of course I've got to keep on trying other options.'

At the start of 1995 he said he believed he had detected a gradual improvement in his condition though nothing dramatic: 'I have lost all my strength and power and I no longer have the balance and stamina I once did – but I don't feel depressed and I don't feel tired. I am determined to go on fighting. I want to be back skiing again.'

## What to expect from a natural therapist

Most natural health practitioners will treat you for the precise way you are feeling at the time you see them.

So, for example, though it is unlikely you will want to see a therapist specifically for a cold or flu you will probably be treated first for that if you turn up for your

appointment with a cold or the start of flu – rather than
the blurred vision or tingling in your fingers you made
the appointment for in the first place.

The principle here is that there is a reason for the
infection and it should be cleared first. Also it may be
linked in some way to the original problem.

You are likely to find this common approach whether
you are seeing an osteopath for your back, a reflexologist
for a hormonal problem, an aromatherapist for relaxation or an acupuncturist for your energy levels. They
will all adjust your treatment for that visit, to encourage
your body to heal itself in the best way possible for you.

Most natural therapists will also encourage you to
'take control' by using terms such as 'taking responsibility for yourself'.

## The significance of 'taking control'

Most natural therapists believe the fact that someone
with a problem has sought out an individual therapist
means that the person wants to take reponsibility for
their own health and is looking for help in actively participating in the process of getting well.

This is very different from the 'allopathic' (conventional medical) principle of treating physical symptoms
in isolation, and using the same remedy for everyone
regardless of physical, mental and emotional differences.
Holistic therapists treat the individual as a complex mixture of interacting influences rather than a 'text-book'
problem requiring text-book solutions.

As most of the case studies described in this book
show, actively participating in your own healing has
been shown to be an important factor in the success of
most natural therapies and that's why a good practitioner will always encourage you to do this, even if it means
just recommending a simple change in lifestyle.

The realization that you can contribute to your own health by small changes in lifestyle can come as a total revelation to many people who have struggled for years with a persistent problem – even one as severe and complex as MS.

For how to find and choose a natural therapist see *Chapter 10*. First, we will look in more detail at the various therapies.

# CHAPTER 7

# Treating your body

*Physical therapies for MS*

This chapter tells you how you can be helped by practitioners using therapies that treat largely the physical aspect of you – though, like most natural therapies, they usually benefit your 'psychological self' as well. The most effective physical therapies for MS are:

- Diet and nutrition
- Exercise and yoga
- Herbal medicine
- Magnet therapy
- Manipulation (Alexander Technique, chiropractic, cranial osteopathy, osteopathy, physiotherapy)
- Massage (and aromatherapy)
- Naturopathy (including hydrotherapy)
- Oxygen therapy (including hyperbaric therapy)

*Note* The aim of the physical therapies is to help the body help itself. Sometimes they are tools you can use on yourself but with treatments such as dietary therapy, herbalism, manipulation and oxygen therapy qualified professional help is *essential*. All have the potential to do great harm in inexperienced hands.

Though most of the therapies listed above have a long history of usefulness few are supported by the sort of scientific research acceptable to most doctors and scientists. They are therefore described as they are *believed* to work by those who use them.

## Diet and nutrition

As we have seen earlier, diet and nutrition have both been shown to play a significant part in MS.

Dietary therapists or dieticians advise on what you should or should not eat while nutritional therapists specialize in recommending therapeutic doses of specific 'food supplements' to treat a condition. For example, in MS they are likely to recommend taking an essential fatty acid such as evening primrose oil.

### Dietary therapy

Treatment by diet involves as much knowing when *not* to eat as what to eat and when. Most specialists in the field will recommend eating a regular amount (as much as you need but no more) of wholesome food, with a good proportion of raw fruit and vegetables, to become and remain healthy. But they will also recommend not eating sometimes.

Though some doctors don't agree, a 24-hour fast is a perfectly safe and highly effective way to help the body fight an infection of any sort if carried out under proper supervision. Fasting helps clear out toxins from the system and leaves the immune system free to concentrate on the healing process.

A trained dietary therapist will also be able to advise on when to eat and what foods work best with other foods, the concept known as 'food combining'. The idea is to help the body 'cleanse' on the one hand and achieve 'optimum nutrition' on the other.

## Jane's story

*Jane, 36, from southern England, found the greatest benefit for her MS came from following an anti-candida diet and having all her mercury amalgam fillings replaced.*

Jane was not diagnosed as having MS until she was 25 but realizes the first symptoms came in her teens.

Nine months after she had her first daughter she had a recurrence of earlier blurred vision, followed by tingling in her arms and legs. Though she feels her doctor and the orthopaedic specialist she saw suspected she had MS because they knew her father had the disease, she herself did not make the link.

In the end it was a neurologist who confirmed the diagnosis after the orthopaedic surgeon told her there was nothing wrong with her: 'The neurologist came straight out with it and I was totally shattered. I said I wanted to fight it but he said he could do nothing and gave me some Valium – he said to help me sleep.'

The specialist told her the MS probably wouldn't affect her for 'five or ten years' and to go ahead and have more children 'if that's what she wanted'. He also told her not to 'waste her time' with self-help methods.

Jane immediately went on the classic MS diet – low fat, evening primrose oil and vitamins, especially vitamin C. She also had hyperbaric oxygen for a year and later had vitamin B12 injections. At the same time she continued seeing the chiropractor she'd been seeing since her days as a competitive gymnast.

She stabilized and this continued for the next six years, during when she 'seriously' investigated food allergies and went on an exclusion diet – 'it was really hard but I stuck at it'. She also saw a doctor who specializes in treating people with MS.

'He recommended I went on an anti-candida diet – no yeast or sugar – and had all my fillings replaced. These are the two things I did that I can say with absolute certainty worked well. I noticed a very definite improvement almost immediately.'

Jane says this improvement became what she calls 'a gradual process of recovery': 'I've restarted HBO, which seems to help, and I'm seeing a very good homoeopath who helps me emotionally. I also swim and exercise regularly. I think it's very important to keep everything working.

'Yoga is good but most is too hard for me now. I'm a great fan of Susie Cornell's exercises [see *Chapter 4*]. They're brilliant but I'm not too good at doing them every day.'

## Nutritional therapy

Nutritional therapy as a discipline in its own right has only really grown up since the Second World War when the idea of concentrating on the food you eat and using concentrated nutrients in a supplement form started in America. Most influential researchers in this field continue to come from America.

Nutritional therapists believe that the immune system can be helped by selecting the right nutrients for a particular person's condition so a consultation with a nutritional therapist is likely to lead to such suggestions as a comprehensive change of diet and, often, the use of supplements or herbs to give the system maximum support.

Few nutritionists these days would accept the official line that the average Western diet contains all the nutrients the body needs. They claim that many sectors of most populations do not get the recommended daily amounts of many essential nutrients at all, either because of poor eating habits or because modern methods of food production make most foods low in nutrients.

The sort of supplements they are likely to recommend for MS are listed in *Chapter 4*.

---

### Allergy testing

Because of the suspected link between food allergies and MS many diet and nutritional therapists will recommend a test for food allergies. The main tests used are:

- Blood testing
- Electrical testing
- Muscle testing or applied kinesiology (AK)
- Pulse testing

The only method regarded as reliable by specialists is blood testing. New tests being developed in America are said to be likely to replace existing techniques – mainly the *cytotoxic test* and the *neutron test* – 'soon'.

None of the other methods are regarded as properly 'scientific' by most doctors because they are either not based on established scientific principles or have not been fully researched.

---

### Exercise and yoga

As explained in *Chapter 4*, keeping muscles working, particularly those affected by MS, is probably the single most important action a sufferer can take to ward off disability. It is important to keep them working to maintain tone, flexibility and strength. In fact it is *not* working them that is more likely to lead to their deterioration than working them.

### Yoga

The ancient Indian technique of yoga is one of the very

best therapies for people with MS, promoting not only physical mobility but mental and emotional calmness.

The Yoga for Health Foundation in Britain claims to have helped more than 3,000 people with MS at the foundation's residential centre, Ickwell Bury, in Bedfordshire, England, with exercises specially designed for sufferers.

'Many who have participated [in the exercise programme] have appreciably improved their physical condition, often holding the improvement,' says the foundation's director Howard Kent. 'An even greater number report an enhanced quality of life and a more positive approach.'

Even though yoga exercises have been proved to benefit every part of the body, right down to the smallest facial muscles, Howard Kent stresses that yoga is very much a 'whole person' approach and so does not recommend physical exercises for MS in isolation from a programme combining mental and emotional exercises as well (see also *Chapter 8*).

---

### Susie's story

*Former model Susie, 43, from Chelmsford, UK, had so much success with special exercise programmes she was taught she has now started teaching others.*

Susie was diagnosed with MS in 1978 whe she was 28 – though she believes her first symptoms started at 17 when she felt what she describes as a sudden 'thumping feeling' in her back when out riding.

Though tests confirmed MS she says the doctors decided not to tell her: 'It was three months before I found out and that was because my then fiancé decided I should know. The doctors said they thought it best I wasn't told.'

'The trouble was when I did know they said there was nothing they could do. They offered me no treatment or counselling of any sort. All they said was I would be in a wheelchair in three months and gave me the address of the MS Society in London for advice on how to get things like wheelchairs and incontinence pads. It was dreadful.'

Feeling constantly tired, weak and depressed, she spent a great deal of time crying. She struggled on this way for most of her 30s: 'I couldn't even manage a shower I was so exhausted all the time. My doctor tried me on steroids but they did no good at all.'

Finally, in 1988 when she was 39, she visited the now world-famous Peto Institute for Conductive Education in Hungry, then unknown in the West. The special exercises she learnt there, developed mainly for people with cerebral palsy, started her on the road to recovery.

'They told me that only 10 per cent of my problem was due to MS; the rest was down to neglect.'

Now realizing there were things she could do for herself after all, she started on a voyage of discovery taking in a range of exercise routines developed by others, including a variety of osteopathic and yogic techniques, and evolved her own programme.

'It's worked for me, I feel fine, and I'd like to help others make it work for them,' she says. 'No one else is doing very much so I feel I must help if I can.'

For more details *see* Appendix A 'MS Under Pressure'.

## Herbal medicine

Herbalism, the use of herbs or plants to heal, is probably the oldest form of medicine known – and was almost the only form of effective medicine in the Western world until recent history.

Traditional herbalists object to modern drugs because they say the process of isolating and extracting specific compounds – which drug companies need to do to 'patent' a drug to make money on it – concentrates the chemicals too much and removes the natural balancing effect of other chemicals in the herb or plant. They also say the body reacts against synthetic chemicals precisely because they are not natural.

Medical herbalism is now enjoying a revival in the West as a result of the unpleasant side-effects of so many synthetic drugs – which people with MS know more about than most – and the arrival of a growing number of practitioners trained in the rich Chinese tradition. This is introducing a whole range of previously unknown and apparently effective remedies for many quite chronic conditions, including MS.

To date, though, the only documented herbs for MS are those from the Western tradition. They include the following.

### Nerve tonics

Oats (can be taken as a tincture or simply as porridge), damiana, skullcap (especially for stress-related problems), vervain, wood betony.

### Nerve relaxants

Black cohosh, black haw, California poppy, chamomile, cramp bark, hops, hyssop, Jamaican dogwood, lady's slipper, lavender, lime blossom, mistletoe, motherwort, Pasque flower, passion flower, rosemary, St John's wort, skullcap and valerian.

*A word of warning* Herbs are powerful drugs and some are dangerous in untrained hands. To make sure you use the right herb in the right dose for the right symptoms, without the risk of side-effects, go only to herbalists who are properly trained and fully qualified (see *Chapter 10* and *Appendix A*).

## Magnet therapy

Research has shown that pulsed electromagnetic fields can promote the healing process, rapidly accelerating the speed of both tissue and bone repair. Based on this evidence some therapists promote the use of magnets as a remedy for any number of conditions, including MS. Benefits from pulsed electromagnetic energy (PEME) are well documented but *not* from wearing the magnetic belts or bandages touted by some.

## Manipulation

Expert manipulation of the body, and especially the bones, muscles and tissues of the spine, has long been said to help a range of persistent long-term (or 'chronic') problems including MS.

### The Alexander Technique

This is a largely self-help technique created earlier this century by F Matthias Alexander, an Australian actor who solved a recurring problem with his breathing and voice when he found that his posture was to blame. The technique is now widely popular with performing artistes of many kinds all over the world.

Alexander established that use affects functioning: in other words, bad postural habits we develop as we get older affect the body's ability to function properly. His technique is a way of learning how to use the body as it was designed to work and how, in most of us, it started out working.

Generally between four and six lessons are needed to correct or 'unlearn' poor postural habits though some people need more.

## Chiropractic

The word 'chiropractic' comes from the Greek and means 'manual practice'. Like osteopathy, chiropractic aims to restore health and 'balance' by manipulation of the bones, muscles and tissues of the body, particularly the spine, so that everything is in its correct place and is working properly.

Unlike osteopaths, though, who consider the main effect is on the blood supply, chiropractors believe it is the nerves that are the important part.

Techniques vary, from the famous bone-cracking 'high velocity thrusts' used by some practitioners to the relatively gentle approach adopted by supporters of the McTimoney method. Chiropractic is generally more vigorous than osteopathy and its practitioners rather more conventionally 'medical' in approach, including using x-rays in their diagnosis.

## Cranial osteopathy

Cranial osteopathy, or the variation known as cranio-sacral therapy, is a method of gently balancing the bones, fluids and membranes of the whole body by the very gentlest manipulation of the bones of the head, especially, and the spine.

Because the bones of the head and spine are attached to the central nervous system and surrounded by fluid (known as the *cerebro-spinal fluid*) the belief is that if the passage of this fluid becomes blocked for any reason, physical or emotional 'dis-ease' occurs.

By placing the hands lightly on the patient's head, back or wherever indicated, and using the softest pressure, the therapist will aim very gently to release these restrictions and restore balance and proper function to the body.

## Osteopathy

Osteopathy – the word means 'bone treatment' – is not just treatment for bones and bad backs even though that is what it is best known for. Osteopathy works to improve the overall structure of the body and its practitioners claim it can benefit almost any disorder, including MS.

Like chiropractic, osteopathy began in America more than 100 years ago and is today so established there that its practitioners are all conventional doctors with a little extra training in manipulation.

Outside America, osteopaths are generally not doctors and train in special colleges. Though the better colleges teach many of the same things as medical schools they put more emphasis on 'naturopathic' techniques such as diet, nutrition and allergy testing – all of which can be useful in the treatment of MS (see also 'Naturopathy' below).

## Physiotherapy

Physiotherapy, or physical therapy in America, is the 'orthodox' equivalent of the other manipulative therapies without their philosophy or claims. In other words, these therapists are professionals within the conventional medical system trained to work to a doctor's instructions to correct and improve a patient's mobility and nothing else.

Some sufferers complain that standard physiotherapy is not particularly helpful or relevant for MS and say they have found greater benefit in the more 'holistic' approach of yoga or specially-designed exercises (see *Chapter 4*).

Others, however, have found benefit from the treatment which, if nothing else, is good at teaching muscle-stretching exercises. Some experts say muscle-stretching is more important in MS than muscle-strengthening.

## Massage

Massage is another of those old but highly effective treatments widely ignored in the West until relatively recently. Whether used as a simple method for relaxing tired and aching muscles and joints or as a more sophisticated therapy, its benefit for a wide range of conditions is now so well recognized that it is in growing use in hospitals and nursing clinics everywhere.

The variations available are enormous, from the quite strong techniques used in Swedish massage to techniques so gentle they hardly seem like massage at all and have more in common with the sort of 'soft tissue' manipulation used by some osteopaths or 'hands-on' healers than anything else.

Its benefit lies in stimulating blood flow to every part of the body, relaxing nerves and in the psychological benefits of feeling 'cared for'.

Two techniques especially therapeutic for MS are massage used in conjunction with aromatic oils (known as 'aromatherapy') and lymph drainage massage.

### Aromatherapy

Aromatherapy treats the body with oils distilled from plants considered to have healing properties. Most of the plants used are well known and are often powerful medicinal herbs (see also *Herbal medicine* above). Such oils are known as 'essential oils'.

Strictly speaking the word 'aromatherapy' means 'smell therapy' and so includes treatment by inhaling, vaporizing and drinking the oils as well as massaging them on. But aromatherapy is almost always taken to mean massaging with aromatic oils these days.

Research has shown that essential oils can help with a wide range of problems, from heart disease to MS. Medical aromatherapist Dr Vivian Lunny, head of research for the UK's Aromatherapy Organizations Council and chairman of the International Federation of Aromatherapy, claims a combination of *palmarosa*, *sandalwood* and *bergamot* is particularly beneficial – though she stresses the need always to tailor the oils to the patient.

They work, she says, essentially by toning and relaxing muscles. This in turn helps restore mobility and general body function. Other combinations can also help with depression and fatigue. Research in France, and to some extent in Britain, has shown that essential oils penetrate the skin, moving into the bloodstream and the lymphatic system within four hours.

According to Dr Lunny, there are both clinical trials and ample case studies to support the use of aromatherapy for MS. But she says it is important to consult a fully-qualified *medical* aromatherapist. Some oils are dangerous, particularly if taken internally or by very young children and pregnant women. A properly-trained therapist should know as much about what oils *not* to take as those *to* take.

### Lymph drainage massage

Lymph drainage massage, or lympathic massage, is a specialized technique offered by some natural therapists to clear toxins from the lymphatic system, a vital part of the body's immune system.

The therapist starts with the nodes in the neck and tries gently to move the fluid by massaging them until the swelling is reduced. It is a safe, simple and sometimes quite dramatically effective treatment.

Another way to stimulate the lymph to move, and one you can do for yourself, is 'dry skin-brushing'. With a long-handled brush, preferably one made of cactus bristle, make long strokes over all skin surfaces toward the centre of the body.

---

**Self-help methods for the lymph system**

- *Diet* Swollen nodes (or glands) are an indication that the system is not working properly. When this happens increase fluids, especially by drinking fennel or fenugreek tea, eating fennel (raw or lightly steamed), or adding sprouting fenugreek seeds to a bowl of raw vegetables. (Processed foods slow the system down.)
- *Exercise* Exercise works as a pump to the lymph, stimulating the fluids to circulate and to be excreted through the bloodstream. Anything that moves the muscles directly is beneficial and one of the best ways for people with MS to do this is swimming.

Another way, MS, even more stimulating, is mini-trampolining or 'rebounding'. Bouncing affects every organ and cell in the body for the better. For a fraction of a second at the top of the bounce the body is weightless, improving the drainage of lymph which in turn speeds elimination of toxins and wastes from the body.

---

## Naturopathy

Naturopathy is the umbrella term now used in most countries to cover a range of therapies coming under the heading of 'natural medicine'. Naturopathy means, literally, natural treatment and its practitioners are generally those trained at specialist colleges in a range of skills that include acupuncture, herbalism, homoeopathy, osteopathy, hydrotherapy, massage, nutrition and diet.

Modern naturopathy has developed out of an earlier very idealistic approach to healing which believed that your body would cure itself of anything as long as you took in only pure air and water, kept clean, indulged in healthy activity and ate the right food. Called 'Nature Cure' or 'Natural Hygiene', it still survives among a few practitioners who think even prescribing vitamin supplements is a corruption.

Except in Britain, naturopathy is becoming the standard training for those interested in practising natural medicine in its widest sense. Countries such as America, Australia, Canada, Germany, Israel, New Zealand and South Africa run full three- to four-year courses leading to a recognized degree of doctor of naturopathy.

Naturopaths – or in Germany, where the idea was first developed last century, *Heilpraktikeren* ('health practitioners') – believe that infections seldom happen if the body is looked after in the way nature intended. But they also believe that getting ill is natural and that methods of cure should follow the same natural principles.

So, far from from being suppressed, symptoms of illness should be encouraged to come out and the body helped and encouraged to fight back and find its proper balance again. Naturopathic therapies effective at treating MS are diet and nutrition, hydrotherapy, and massage (see relevant sections in this chapter).

Naturopaths will also routinely encourage brief fasting to get over simple infections such as flu and pay a great deal of attention to the health of the bowels (intestines) where nutrients are absorbed into the bloodstream.

This has particular relevance for people with MS because of the theory that bacterial toxins in the gut may have a part to play in the cause of MS (see *Chapter 3*). For this reason many naturopaths encourage special diets to clear the gut and eliminate the overgrowth of unfriendly fungi and bacteria that can colonize the intestines and, according to naturopaths, contribute to toxicity, allergy and poor immunity.

Some naturopaths even make use of a special treatment for washing the gut clean called colonic irrigation, or colon hydrotherapy (see *box*).

---

### Colonic irrigation

Colonic irrigation, or colonic hydrotherapy, is a sort of 'internal bath' that involves inserting a small hose-like device with two tubes into the rectum. One of the tubes pumps water in and the other draws it out again.

It is far more drastic an operation than a simple enema (which most people can perform on themselves quite easily and simply) and not without risks and dangers. Practitioners need to be skilled as well as knowledgeable and a high degree of hygiene is vital.

There is no evidence colonic irrigation can help MS but that is certainly the claim of some naturopaths.

---

### Hydrotherapy

Hydrotherapy is water therapy and is another of those simple yet highly effective therapies with a tradition stretching back beyond human records. Any form of therapy with water is hydrotherapy and one of the best known, and most effective in MS, is swimming (see *Chapter 4*). But some sufferers claim that special baths also help. Two types said to be beneficial are:

- cold baths (see *page 43*)
- hydrogen peroxide baths (see *'Oxygen therapies'* over).

## Oxygen therapies

A number of therapies make use of oxygen's unique life-giving properties and are said to be effective for MS. They include the following.

### Hyperbaric oxygen therapy

Hyperbaric oxygen therapy (HBO) involves sitting inside a special sealed chamber at twice the normal atmospheric pressure while breathing in pure oxygen through a mask, so forcing more oxygen into the bloodstream (see *figure 9*). An individual session normally lasts about an hour and a course of treatment 20 days.

Oxygen is a natural free radical 'scavenger' (see *page 34*) and the treatment is said to accelerate repair of tissue, especially brain and blood vessels. In Italy it is a standard treatment for stroke victims and in many countries it is now commonly also used in the treatment of MS.

Most UK doctors don't believe HBO helps MS but the therapy is officially supported by the Federation of Multiple Sclerosis Therapy Centres in the UK which claims that well over a million treatments have been carried out successfully over the last ten years without any problem.

The federation says that though HBO is not a cure it is an effective preventive measure that has shown consistent benefits for sufferers, particularly in controlling and improving bladder function.

The main criticism of the technique outside its use for MS is that, like steroids, it goes for short-term gain at long-term expense. Too much oxygen too quickly can produce intense energy but it also accelerates the ageing process.

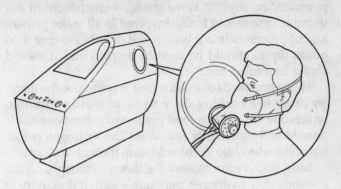

**Fig. 9 A modern hyperbaric therapy unit**

*Hydrogen peroxide*

Better known as a bleach and disinfectant, hydrogen peroxide ($H_2O_2$) is, in fact, a fast and efficient anti viral agent as well as being antibacterial and antifungal. Its use in therapy was developed in America in the 1950s and 1960s where it found fame in the treatment of candidiasis and arthritis.

Treatment is normally either by drinking very dilute amounts of special 'food grade' $H_2O_2$ or by taking supplements or by injection. By injection, or *intravenous infusion*, the treatment can only be done by a doctor. An alternative to hydrogen peroxide, and the preferred option for some practitioners when taken orally (by mouth) is magnesium peroxide ($MgO_2$).

Alwyne Pilsworth, director of the Oxygen Therapy Information Centre in Britain, says some success has been recorded for the therapy with MS, particularly in America, but he stresses treatment should only be under expert guidance.

'There are no recorded cases of adverse effects from ingestion or infusion of the correct doses of hydrogen peroxide,' he says. 'It is the chemical component of our immune system and is also involved in all major physiological processes in our bodies. But only 35 per cent food grade liquid should be used in therapy and it should *always* be diluted first.'

He recommends one of the best ways to use the therapy in MS is by taking daily baths of tepid water into which one cup of 35% food grade hydrogen peroxide is poured and thoroughly stirred in. The hydrogen peroxide is absorbed into the bloodstream through the skin.

Most doctors are against the therapy, though, on the grounds that hydrogen peroxide's antiviral activity is short-lived and, more seriously, it can damage cell membranes and accelerate free radical activity in the body.

## Ozone therapy

Popular in Germany, and increasingly so now in other parts of the world, the therapy involves 'pepping' up blood by injecting ozone. Ozone is, effectively, 'super oxygen' $(O_3)$. It is present naturally in the air – you can sometimes smell it after a thunderstorm for example – but in therapy it is created artificially by a special device that gives oxygen $(O_2)$ an extra molecule.

Ozone is a strong 'energizer' as well as having known anti viral, anti bacterial and anti fungal properties. Interestingly, one of the viruses it is most effective against is the *Herpes zoster* virus that some experts consider might be a trigger for MS (see *Chapter 3*).

The treatment involves drawing blood off, passing it through an 'ozonator' and re-infusing it into the body, a procedure that usually takes about 20 minutes. It can only be carried out by a doctor. An alternative method popular in America is squirting humidified ozone into the rectum. A 30-second burst is said to produce about half a litre (1 pint) of ozone and it is better absorbed into the bloodstream this way than by the injection method.

But though specialists use the treatment for MS, it has not been proven yet in clinical trials and the American Food and Drug Administration (FDA) is currently investigating it for safety.

# CHAPTER 8

# Treating your mind and emotions

*Psychological therapies for* MS

The effect of our mind and emotions on how we feel physically is well known and documented – but has this any relevance in a condition such as MS? The answer is a most emphatic yes.

MS is a disease that can have profound psychological effects at every stage, and it is now known that in the later stages MS can also affect mental faculties such as memory and concentration.

### How psychological therapies help physical disease

When you feel good it may be partly to do with the fact your body is making *endorphins*, just one of the many chemicals known as *hormones* made by the *endocrine system*.

Hormones control a great deal of our basic behaviour, especially our moods. They are the vital link between what we think and feel and our physical health. They are a sort of 'switching station' between the two. That's how physical factors not only affect how we think and feel – affect us psychologically, that is – but how we think and feel also affects us physically.

So psychological factors may be just as important reasons for infection taking a hold in you as physical factors. In simple terms it amounts to the fact that when you feel low, 'negative' hormones triggered by such feelings depress your immune system and slow down its response.

But it is a cycle that can be broken. You may want and need the help of others in this process and in that case this chapter tells you some of the many ways available to help you.

## Affirmations

Put simply, an affirmation is thinking yourself well. Perhaps the best known affirmation is that invented by the French chemist and hypnotist Emile Coué more than a century ago: 'Every day, in every way, I am getting better and better.'

Repeated 15 to 20 times twice a day, morning and night, it has helped people with many seemingly hopeless problems, including invalids.

Medically speaking an affirmation is *auto-suggestion*. It is a central feature of many forms of meditation such as a Western version known as *autogenics* and Oriental systems like *transcendental meditation* or 'TM' (*see* 'Meditation').

Probably the best known affirmations today are those by the American therapist Louise Hay. In her book *Heal Your Body* (Eden Grove, US, 1989) and *You Can Heal Your Life* (Eden Grove, US, 1988), with its affirmations on every page, she identifies a number of negative thought-patterns and beliefs, and teaches you how to understand the effect these have on your life.

Using complementary techniques like *relaxation* and *visualization* with affirmations she has helped many people change from negative ways to more positive ones.

## Relaxation

The fact that so many therapists now actively encourage and teach relaxation shows just how far most of us have moved from a state in which relaxation is seen as natural and normal and how much so many people need to rediscover it.

Of course some relaxation happens automatically – when you have a bath perhaps. But you can reach that state without getting wet with the help of a few simple exercises, many of which you can teach yourself from the books now available (see *Appendix B*).

For example, simply stretching and breathing deeply can be very relaxing (as in yawning and sighing). Relaxing the body totally by making a conscious effort may not seem so simple but it can be done quite quickly with the right instruction and practice.

The British Holistic Medical Association (see *Appendix A*) publishes audio-tapes for relaxation as part of its *Tapes for Health* series.

## Visualization

This is a technique which uses the power of the mind – in this case, your imagination – to affect your body for the better. It has been used in many countries in the treatment of cancer though results are variable, depending it seems very much on the personality and character of the person doing the imagining or 'visualizing'.

Against MS, for example, the sufferer could imagine a winged angel or a bird flying through his or her nervous system collecting up all the damaged cells and replacing them with fresh, healthy cells.

Visualization can be a particularly useful method for children and young people who tend to have much freer and more vivid imaginations than adults and so achieve much more positive results.

But adults can achieve good results too if they let

---

### A simple relaxation exercise

Sit in a comfortable position somewhere (it is better not to lie down or you are liable to fall asleep if the exercise is successful!). Starting with your feet, wiggle your toes. Then squeeze your feet and let them go. Rotate your ankles, and feel the difference. Then do the same with your calves, knees and thighs.

Clench your buttocks and relax them. Tighten the stomach muscles, slowly breathe in and then more slowly breathe out. When you reach your shoulders hunch them up and release (many people hold tension in their shoulders without realizing it). Do this a few times. Finish by screwing your face up and stretching your jaw before releasing. Relax. You should feel quite relaxed.

See if you can keep this feeling of relaxation during the course of the day. Test your body from time to time. If you think you've tensed up run through the sequence again. It doesn't take long – no more than a few minutes – and is easy to fit into even the busiest routine. With practice you'll find it will help you cope better and give you more stamina and clarity of mind.

---

themselves. Imagine yourself somewhere where you feel happy and content and gradually become part of the scene. See yourself without illness or distress and visualize yourself fit and well with healthy limbs and a cheerful outlook.

At its best it is a mild form of self-hypnosis and at its worst a pleasant, and therefore probably relaxing, diversion. Either way it can have benefits.

### Biofeedback

Not exactly 'natural', in the sense that it uses simple technology, biofeedback is nonetheless an extremely safe, gentle and very effective way of helping your psychological condition.

It uses a meter to help you recognize how your body is behaving at any given moment from fine electrodes held either in the hand or connected to a band tied around your head. For example, the meter will register one reading when you are tense and another when you are relaxed.

By using the meter to monitor the physical effects produced by specific feelings you gradually learn, with the help of a trained therapist, how to influence your responses and so educate your body to do more of what helps you and less of what hurts.

## Counselling therapies

As the name implies, counselling therapies generally encourage you to sit quietly and talk about yourself and your problems to a trained and experienced listener who will help you express your feelings, find insights and see solutions for yourself.

### Counselling
Counselling is becoming such a well-organized, regulated and widespread therapy these days it is wrong to call it unconventional any longer. A clearly safe and gentle approach, counselling is an extremely important and effective way of helping many people cope with major periods of stress and strain, including occasional consequences of MS such as a broken marriage, redundancy, debt or a sense of sexual inadequacy.

In Britain and America it is increasingly common to find professional counsellors at conventional health centres and clinics.

### Psychotherapy
Like standard counselling, psychotherapy is a method of allowing people to talk through emotional and mental problems and receive support and guidance for them.

But psychotherapy, as the name implies, concentrates more on tackling the deeper, often hidden, underlying causes of disease.

It does this by trying to get people to understand and face up to psychological problems within themselves by talking them through with a trained listener. This can be done on either an individual basis or as part of a group.

*Psychotherapy has little to do with psychiatry which is a purely medical discipline based largely on drug treatment of mental problems.*

There is an enormous variety of psychological therapies available – far more than there is room to list here – and they cover almost every type and style of approach, from the spiritually complex such as psychosynthesis to the down-to-earth like laughter therapy.

Other psychological therapies you are likely to come across are art therapy, co-counselling (or re-evaluation counselling), encounter therapy, Gestalt therapy, humanistic psychology, Jungian or analytic psychology, music or sound therapy, drama therapy, bioenergetics, psychoanalysis (Freudian psychotherapy), Rogerian therapy, transpersonal psychology and transactional analysis.

There are also growing numbers of therapists, including doctors, who specialize in 'stress management' and often they will be in the best position to guide you towards the right psychological approach if they can't help you themselves (see *Appendix A*).

### Flower remedies

Flower remedies – the most famous being the 'Bach remedies' named after British homoeopath Dr Edward Bach who devised them earlier this century – treat physical conditions by treating the psychological problems it is believed lie behind them.

Dr Bach, for example, convinced that a negative outlook affects both the body and events in our lives as well as the way we face up to them, developed a set range of 38 remedies for every type of human emotion, from anger to vulnerability. Each is intended to treat the individual rather than the illness he or she is suffering from (see also *Chapter 9*).

## Hypnotherapy

Hypnotherapy, or hypnosis, is a very specific form of therapy, well supported by research, in which trained specialists – and they may be doctors as well as non-medical practitioners – aim to help you deal with unconscious or subconscious mental and emotional problems.

This is normally done by getting you into a state of deep relaxation to help you 'get in touch with' the cause or causes of the distress or to imagine ways in which you could cope more easily.

Once this is known it may be easier to deal with it consciously through standard counselling or psychotherapy. Some hypnotherapists are also counsellors or psychotherapists.

Hypnotherapy is also a way of learning to relax deeply. The many 'subliminal' tapes now on the market use a form of hypnosis to aid relaxation although some therapists have voiced concerns about their use without professional supervision.

Though stage hypnotists have given hypnotism a bit of a bad name, hypnotherapy is a genuinely helpful technique. But because it is such a very powerful form of therapy clearly open to abuse it is important to check out a therapist very thoroughly before going to one. *Chapter 10* tells you how to do this. The alternative is to find a doctor who specializes in hypnosis (see *Appendix A*).

## Meditation

When the mind is at rest it has, like the body, a much greater capacity for healing itself. Meditation is a way of resting your mind beyond simply thinking nothing or 'day-dreaming'. It has been best described as 'passive concentration' or 'active attention'.

There is a wide variety of techniques, some promoted by religious organizations which make quite large claims, but there is, or should be, nothing mystical or mysterious about meditation. It is not a religion and you don't have to sit in the well-known 'lotus' position, with your eyes closed.

There is good evidence that meditation, as well as supporting your immune system, lowers levels of stress and brings on a strong sense of peace and tranquillity

In Holland people who practise transcendental meditation can now get lower health insurance premiums because it has been shown to lower blood pressure and so lead to fewer heart and circulation problems.

Anyone can meditate but it takes a bit of practice to do it properly which is why it is quite a good idea to be shown how to do it by someone experienced. The basic idea is to relax the body and then try and do the same with the mind. This can be difficult at first but with practice it becomes easier.

A well-known way to make it easier is to repeat, silently or aloud, a single word or phrase over and over again. This word is called a *mantra* in Eastern meditational practice. The sound should be pleasing and your mind should become focused on it to the exclusion of everything else. An alternative is to fix your gaze on a single object such as a candle or stone.

Some tips. Don't lie down or you could fall asleep. Sit upright in a comfortable and well-supported position. And don't worry about stray thoughts that flit through your mind and don't worry about how well you may be doing. The most important thing is to adopt a 'let it all happen' approach.

The process of meditation should be easy. Experienced meditators say: 'Don't push the river: let it flow by itself.'

### Autogenic training

A Westernized rediscovery of the basic principles of Eastern meditation, autogenics was created more than half a century ago by a German psychiatrist and hypnotist Dr Johannes Schultz.

Autogenics makes use of six standard exercises that involve directing your attention inwards and focusing your mind on phrases relating to different parts of the body. You become 'awake' to

- sensations of heaviness in your body
- warmth in your arms and legs
- your calm and regular heartbeat
- your easy and natural breathing
- warmth in your abdomen
- coolness in your head

Under trained supervision, usually from doctors, these purely mental exercises are introduced gradually at weekly individual or small group training sessions over an eight-week period. The patients then practise in a comfortable, stable sitting position or lying down. Like most conventional medication it is 'taken' three times daily ten minutes after meals!

### Yoga

As already explained in *Chapter 7*, yoga is one of the most complete mind–body therapies there is and has been shown to have powerful benefits in MS, involving as it does effective movement with an equally effective mental approach that can have profound psychological benefits.

For maximum results yoga is one of those therapies best learnt at first hand from a good instructor rather than from a book or video, at least in the first place. These days yoga is so well known and widespread it is fairly easy to find classes.

# CHAPTER 9

# Treating your 'life force'

*'Subtle energy' therapies for helping MS*

A number of therapies encourage the body to 'recharge its batteries' by stimulating not just physical energy – the sort of energy you can get from eating the right foods for example – but what is called 'subtle' energy. This is energy said to exist at a subtle or invisible level: that is, it is 'sub-atomic' or 'psychic'. Another term commonly used instead of subtle energy is 'life force'. Examples of subtle energy or life force therapies are acupuncture, homoeopathy and healing.

Because 'life force' has so far eluded measurement, proof of its existence remains inconclusive and controversial: some people swear by it while others say it is all fantasy. But acupuncture, homoeopathy and healing have not only a long history of success and scientific studies to back them up but are also used regularly by a growing number of doctors.

There is no clinical proof that any energy therapy can help MS specifically but evidence from sufferers suggests that the energy therapies most *likely* to be helpful are those here.

### Acupuncture

Acupuncture originated in China more than 4,000 years ago. The earliest books on the subject appeared around 475BC.

Today there are estimated to be some three million practitioners worldwide. Most of them are in the Far East but a growing number are now in the West where doctors as well as physio (or physical) therapists are looking increasingly to acupuncture for the successful treatment of pain relief and addictions. Western hospitals, too, have started using acupuncture as an anaesthetic where drugs are not appropriate or possible.

The treatment uses very fine gold, silver or steel needles – so fine most people don't even feel them being inserted – to stimulate the body's subtle energy (known as *qi* or *chi* in Chinese) at any one or more of some 361 specific points situated along the 14 'meridians' or energy pathways said to run through the body (see *figure 10*). This process is believed to balance out the flow of subtle energy in the body and so help the natural self-healing tendency.

A variation is the technique known as *moxibustion* in which a gentle heat is applied to an energy point using *moxa*, a dried powdered herb (usually common mugwort). This is either attached to the needle so that the heat transfers down the needle to the energy point or it is rolled into small cones and slowly burnt over the point on top of a protective covering. Sometimes a few cones are used together. The belief is that this 'draws' and 'heats' the energy making more energy available.

Acupuncture and herbs are often used together in China and throughout the Orient and this combined practice is known collectively as Traditional Chinese Medicine (TCM). The list of herbs used in Chinese medicine is vast and practitioners of TCM in the West tend to be Chinese. Western practitioners seem to prefer to concentrate mainly on acupuncture and moxibustion.

## Vicky's story

*Hospital manager Vicky has found homoeopathy, reflex therapy and exercise help her MS best.*

Physiotherapist-turned-hospital manager Vicky, 39, was diagnosed with MS when she was 32, three years after an attack that left her right side numb.

Tests for a suspected disc problem proved negative and when the symptoms went Vicky thought nothing of it for another two years – until she woke one day with a feeling as if a tight belt had been tied around her.

'When the specialist said he thought it was MS I felt relief,' says Vicky. 'At last it had a name – and that meant I could start doing something about it.' But not until a severe attack at 34 that put her out of action for five months was she spurred into action.

She went to her local MS therapy centre and though she rejected the hyperbaric oxygen therapy offered – 'I didn't like the thought of being stuck in that chamber for an hour' – she immediately went on a low-fat diet, started taking evening primrose oil and went on a regular exercise programme.

She also saw a homoeopathic doctor. 'He was brilliant,' says Vicky. 'He tested me and found I was allergic to lead, mercury and aluminium.'

She was put on a special course of homoeopathic remedies, including *sulphur*, *nux vomica* and *rhus tox*, and had all her mercury amalgam fillings replaced. Her homoeopath also prescribed the herb *ginseng* for more energy and vitamin B12 for tissue repair.

'Homoeopathy made a very definite improvement. I felt well again for the first time. It has helped me more than anything,' she says.

Another treatment she says has helped and still has regularly is reflex therapy, a gentle form of reflexology: 'It definitely helps and I feel great after it.'

She also practises a form of Oriental movement known as *t'ai chi chu'an* and swims regularly as well as doing her own programme of muscle-stretching exercises. 'Stretching muscles is even more important than strengthening them,' she says.

A second severe attack in 1994, when she was 38, involving her in a lot of pain, led Vicky to have her first course of steroids. It got rid of the pain and allowed her to get back to work.

But she still believes that taking responsibility for her own care and trying a wide range of alternative treatments is the best way forward.

'Conventional medicine is really rather bewildered by MS and manages it badly so I think it is important patients look around and try and find what works best for them'.

## Cupping

A less well-known variation of TCM beginning to gain a following in the West is the art of 'cupping'. Cupping is the use of small jars or cups (usually glass) to stimulate and 'draw' the body's energy points in much the same way as needles.

A lighted taper is held inside the jar and then quickly removed to create a vacuum so that the jar clamps itself to the body and 'sucks' on the point. The cup is left in place for perhaps ten minutes for full effect. For local congestion and inflammation cupping is often used with needles.

A Western version of cupping is known as 'Vacuflex'. It uses a small pump to create the vacuum and a number of different-sized suction pads. It is claimed to be quicker and more effective than the manual version.

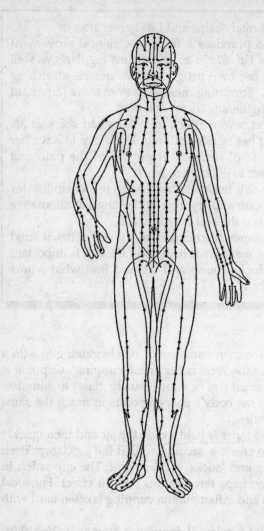

**Fig. 10 The acupuncture 'energy' meridians**

## Acupressure

Acupressure is a widely-used and popular form of therapy which uses finger pressure (and sometimes elbow, knee or heel pressure) on the same points of the body as in acupuncture. This is why it is often called 'acupuncture without needles'. Some people believe it may even have been an earlier form of acupuncture or a variation developed for those who didn't have or didn't like needles.

The principles are the same as in acupuncture but most modern forms in use today were developed not in China but Japan. The best known variation is *shiatsu* ('shiatsu' means 'finger pressure' in Japanese) but other names are *do-in*, *jin shen* (or *shin*) and *shen tao*.

## Healing

Healing – better known by most people as 'faith healing' or 'spiritual healing' – is probably the simplest, safest and most natural of all methods of healing in that it involves nothing but the touch, or sometimes only the thoughts, of the healer to work (though healers themselves usually say there is a lot more to healing than simply placing your hands on someone and hoping for the best!).

Whether the healing is caused by the healer, some mysterious 'force' that is channeled through them or simply the body's own healing powers being stimulated and reinforced, healing has been shown to work for many people. It is certainly not to be scoffed at and is worth trying if you are so inclined.

### Therapeutic touch

Therapeutic touch or TT is a modern version of healing by the laying-on-of-hands. The term is used in countries, particularly the United States, where to call yourself a 'healer' and to claim to heal by, in effect, psychic or supernatural means, is illegal in many states.

In spite of this TT is based on the belief in the actual transfer of energy from the person touching to the person being touched and is in common and increasing use by nurses in clinics and hospitals in America.

## Homoeopathy

Made widely famous and popular in Britain by its use by the Royal Family, homoeopathy suffers from no explanation acceptable to scientists of why and how it works. But there are now a number of trials that appear to show that it does work – and a growing number of doctors are now specializing in it.

Homoeopathy is a 'complete' or self-contained system of medicine developed some 200 years ago by a German doctor called Samuel Hahnemann based on early Greek principles of medicine. Hahnemann discovered by treating himself that a very small amount of what causes a disease also cures it. This gave rise to his principle of 'like cures like' and that remains the basis of homoeopathy to this day.

Homoeopathic remedies are made by taking only the smallest amounts of a specific substance, usually from plants or minerals, diluting them in water with a little alcohol and shaking them vigorously. This vigorous shaking, known as *succussion*, is central to how homoeopathy is said to work.

The process of diluting and shaking is done several times. Unlike most conventional doctors, who believe that the higher the concentration of something the stronger it is, homoeopaths believe the remedy gets more potent each time it is diluted and shaken – hence the term *potentization* to describe the process.

Homoeopathic remedies are usually given as small

white tablets on to which the potentized mixture has been dripped.

Homoeopaths, like most natural therapists, usually see physical symptoms of disease as something deeper and they will always want to see a patient personally and take a detailed history to get to the bottom of what they think is wrong before prescribing. That's why self-prescribing is not recommended by most homoeopaths.

Homoeopathy is widely available in most countries outside North America (some American states have banned its practice) and in Britain it is the oldest natural therapy available free on the National Health Service through doctors qualified as homoeopaths. A derivative of homoeopathy is flower remedies.

## Flower remedies

Flower remedies (see also *Chapter 8*) use the 'essences' of certain flowers to treat the underlying psychological causes of disease.

The original flower remedies were devised in the 1920s and 1930s by a British homoeopath, Dr Edward Bach, and though plant-based are more homoeopathic than herbal in the way they are said to work. In other words they act psychologically and psychically rather than chemically.

The main problem with the many flower remedies now being sold, including varieties from both America and Australia, is that because of this unique psychological–psychic combination no one has so far explained scientifically how they might work and no trials have taken place to prove they do what they claim.

Nevertheless the fact remains that whether or not the effect is purely 'placebo' (you get well because you believe it and for no other reason) flower remedies are used extensively throughout the world by many thousands of people who swear by their benefit.

**Examples of Bach flower remedies for MS**

| | |
|---|---|
| Cherry plum | For tension, fear, uncontrolled or irrational thought |
| Crab apple | For shame at the ailment |
| Gorse | For feelings of hopelessness, defeatism and pessimism |
| Mustard | For a 'dark cloud' descending, feeling sad and low for no reason |
| Olive | For exhaustion, feeling drained of energy |
| Rock rose | For feeling suddenly alarmed or scared |
| Sweet chestnut | For dejection and despair |
| Willow | For resentfulness and bitterness, and always thinking 'poor me' |
| 'Rescue Remedy' | A combination of five remedies (cherry plum, clematis, impatiens, rock rose and Star of Bethlehem) for shock, illness, grief, injury or trauma |

## Reflexology

Reflexology, or sometimes reflex therapy, is simply described as foot massage but therapists say it is more than this. Said to be a modern revival of a healing method widely practised in the ancient world, reflexology probably has links with acupressure and acupuncture.

In Britain it has been recognized by the Chartered Society of Physiotherapists, the official national body for physiotherapists, since 1993.

Like both acupressure and acupuncture, reflexology is based on the idea that lines of energy run through the body and these lines link all the major organs to specific 'reflex' points in the feet. According to reflexologists the bottom of each foot can be 'mapped' with areas or 'zones' which correspond to these various organs (see *figure 11*) and the organs can be affected by putting the reflex points under pressure.

Pressure is usually applied by using the thumb and fingers. No pain means no problem – but any sort of discomfort or pain is said to indicate a problem in the corresponding area of the body and pressure is applied to the painful point. Sometimes this is distinctly uncomfortable but by working on the point for a few moments the pain usually eases and a response is felt in the affected organ.

So, for example, a headache might be relieved by having pressure applied to the base of the big toe (which corresponds to the base of the neck) and congested lungs by pressing the ball of the foot.

Reflex therapy is a version using much gentler pressure.

Reflexology does not claim to be able to remove inflammation or infection once it is there but therapists claim treatment can speed recovery and help maintain it. Most patients say the therapy has a strongly relaxing effect and this will improve circulation and benefit most bodily functions whether it helps individual organs or not. Some evidence of its relaxing qualities is the fact that many people say they feel like resting or sleeping after a treatment.

A modern 'high-tech' version of reflexology called 'Vacuflex' has recently been introduced from Denmark and South Africa. It claims to achieve better results more quickly by using special felt boots and a system of suction pads. Air is drawn out of the boots by a pump and the feet given an 'all-over' squeeze from the vacuum that results. The suction pads are then used in much the same way as 'cupping' (see *page 105*) to stimulate various reflex points on the feet, legs, arms and hands.

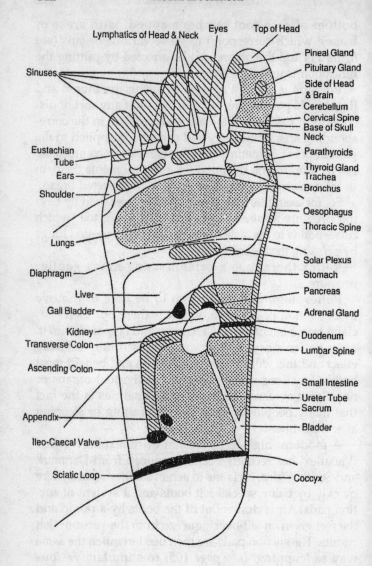

**Fig. 11 Reflex 'zones' on the right foot**

## Other subtle energy therapies

Among many therapies claiming to help almost any illness, including MS, by influencing the body's 'life force' or subtle energy are *crystal* or *gem therapy*, *Aura-Soma* oils and *radionics*. In the case of oils, crystals and gems the colour is said to be as important as the 'vibration' of the gem, crystal or oil.

Though there is good scientific evidence that some colours can affect mood and therefore help by aiding relaxation there is, as yet, no published research of any sort, either scientific or anecdotal (based on case histories), that proves any of the above therapies can do what they claim.

But crystals and coloured oils certainly look good and if they work – and some clearly do for some people – it is as likely to be because patients feel relaxed and confident as a result of believing in what is happening as anything else.

This is still a form of healing, though, and if the result is a reduction in suffering, for whatever reason and to whatever degree, it cannot be altogether dismissed.

What is important here is that the person carrying out the therapy seems to be as, or even more, important as the method they use. Like the healers or shamans of old – and as many a modern doctor knows only too well – belief in the therapist is often the only trigger needed for a person to feel better.

For how to find and choose a good therapist turn to the next chapter.

# CHAPTER 10

# How to find and choose a natural therapist

*Tips and guidelines for finding reliable help*

It is much easier now to find the right therapist than it was even a few years ago – but it is still not easy enough. The sheer variety of therapies is bewildering in itself and in many countries natural therapists are still not fully organized. There is no shortage of directories and advertisements but it's difficult to assess the reliability of their information. So how do you find a therapist you can trust?

### Starting the search: local sources

As we have seen, many of the natural therapies highlighted in this book have their roots in antiquity. Some have existed for as long as human beings have lived on Earth, and finding a good practitioner has been a matter of tuning in to the community 'bush telegraph'. Word of mouth is still the best way to find the right practitioner.

Speak to anyone whose opinion you respect, especially a fellow sufferer. (You will also want to know who should be avoided, and which therapies might not help you at all.) If this does not work there are several other ways you can try.

### Doctors' clinics and medical centres

If you need help urgently you must see your family doctor. It has already been explained in this book that your condition can decline quickly without the proper treatment. If you ask about natural therapies at your first appointment, be prepared to hear anything from a dire warning to a recommendation that you might try a natural therapist once your condition is stable.

### Natural health centres

Your nearest natural health centre should be happy to advise you. Your first impressions will often be a good guide to the quality of service they provide. Are the staff well informed and friendly? Is the place clean and comfortable? Does the atmosphere make you feel comfortable from the moment you walk in? It should. It matters. You are bringing them your trust and your custom and both should be treated with the utmost respect.

A good centre should have plenty of information explaining the therapies and introducing the practitioners. In a well-run practice the receptionist or owner will know all about the different therapies on offer. It's a bad sign if they don't.

You may still be unsure after your first impressions whether to book in or not. If so, ask to meet the person who might be treating you, just to test the waters. This should be possible, even in a busy practice.

Don't start off by telling your full life history, but some practices do offer you this opportunity during a free consultation – usually 15 minutes – just to see whether you have come to the right place or not.

### Local practitioners

Practitioners tend to know who's who in the area, even in therapies other than their own. So if you know, say, a reflexologist, but want a homoeopath, ask for a recommendation. The same applies if you know a practitioner

socially and so don't want to consult him or her profes-
sionally. Practitioners are usually happy to recommend
someone else in the same field.

### Healthfood stores and alternative bookshops

The staff in these kinds of shops often have a good local
knowledge as well as an interest in the subject of natural
therapies. The shop may well have a noticeboard with
local practitioners' business cards on it. Remember,
though, the most experienced and well-established practitioners don't need this kind of advertising, so you
might miss them altogether if you don't actually check
up by asking.

### Other sources of local knowledge

Don't forget that your local pharmacist often has contacts with both conventional and natural therapists. The
local library or information centre may be another good
source of contact, especially for finding self-help or support groups.

Computers (using a modem) can provide information
via the Internet system and other sources worth trying
are health farms, beauty therapists and citizens' advice
bureaux.

## Wider sources of information

If you have no luck on a local level, don't give up – there
are several more leads you can follow up at a national
level.

### 'Umbrella' organizations

The natural therapies are increasingly coming together
under 'umbrella' organizations that represent a therapy
or range of therapies nationally under one banner or
heading. These national umbrella organizations have
lists of registered and approved practitioners, and in the

case of the more established therapies (such as chiropractic) have their own regulatory bodies already in place.

It is better to phone than to write or fax because this should give you a good idea of how well organized the group is. You may find that the group you are contacting has several different associations under its banner. A small charge may be made for each association's register but if you can afford it get the lot and then make up your own mind.

*Newspapers, magazines and local directories*
Many therapists advertise. If you find local practitioners this way it's a good idea to talk to them and check them out first.

## Checking professional organizations

Some organizations are genuine groups that really keep a check on their members, while others seem to spring up like weeds, apparently interested only in collecting membership fees and giving themselves credibility. This section helps you do your own weeding.

*Why do professional organizations exist?*
The purposes of governing bodies for natural therapies are:

- to keep up-to-date lists of their members so you can check whether someone is really on their list
- to protect you by making sure that their members are fully trained, licensed and insured against accident, negligence and malpractice
- to give you someone to complain to if you are unhappy with any aspect of treatment you have received, and you can't sort the matter out with your therapist
- to protect their members by giving good ethical and legal advice

- to represent their members when laws which might affect them are being made
- to work towards improvements in education for their members both before and after qualifying
- to work towards greater awareness of the benefit of each therapy in conventional medical circles
- to improve public awareness of the benefit of each therapy

*Questions to ask professional organizations*

A good organization will publish clear and simple information on its status and purposes along with its membership list. As they don't all do this you may find it useful to contact them again on receiving your list to ask the following:

- When was the association founded? (You may be reassured to hear it has been around for 50 years. If the association is new, however, don't reject it out of hand. Ask why it was formed – it may be innovative.)
- How many members does it have? (Size reflects public demand, as few therapists could survive in a therapy if there was no call for it. The bigger organizations generally have a better track record and greater public acceptance, but a small association may just reflect the fact that the therapy is very specialized or still in its infancy – not necessarily a bad thing.)
- When was the therapy that it represents started?
- Is it a charity or educational trust – with a proper constitution, management committee, and published accounts – or is it a private limited company? (Charities have to be non-profitmaking, work in the public interest, and be open to inspection at any time. Private companies don't.)
- Is it part of a larger network of organizations? (If so, this implies it is interested in progress by consensus with other groups, and not just in furthering its own

aims. By and large, groups that go their own way are more suspect than those that join in.)

- Does the organization have a code of ethics (upholding standards of professional behaviour) and disciplinary procedures? If so, what are they?
- How do its members gain admission to its register? Is it linked to only one school? (Beware of associations whose heads are also head of the school they represent: unbiased help may be in short supply with this type of 'one man band'.)
- Do members have to have proof of professional indemnity insurance? This should cover:
  - accidental damage to yourself or your property while you are on the practitioner's work premises
  - negligence (either the failure of the practitioner to exercise the 'duty of care' owed to you, or his or her falling below the standards of clinical competence demanded by his or her qualifications, bringing about an overall worsening of your problem)
  - malpractice (a 'falling from grace' over professional conduct, involving, for example, dishonesty, sexual misconduct or breach of confidence – your personal details should *never* be discussed with a third person without your permission)

## Checking training and qualifications

If you have reassured yourself so far but are still puzzled by what the training actually involves, ask a few more questions:

- How long is the training?
- Is it full or part time?
- If it is part time but shorter than a full-time course leading to the same qualifications, does the time spent at lectures and in clinic add up to the same as a full-time course overall? (In other words, is it a short cut?)

- Does it include seeing patients under supervision at a college clinic and in real practices?
- What do the initials after the therapist's name mean? Do they denote simply membership of an organization or do they indicate in-depth study?
- Are the qualifications recognized? If so, by whom? (This is becoming more relevant as the therapy organizations group together and start to form state-recognized registers in many countries. But the really important thing to know is if the qualifications are recognized by an independent outside assessment authority.)

### Making the choice

Making the final choice is a matter of using a combination of common sense and intuition, and finding the resolution to give someone a try. Don't forget that the most important part of the whole process is your resolve to feel better, to have more control over your state of health, and hopefully to see an improvement in your condition. The next most important part is that you feel comfortable with your chosen therapist.

### What is it like seeing a natural therapist?

Since most natural therapists, even in those countries with state health systems, still work privately, there is no established common pattern.

Although they may all share more or less a belief in the principles outlined in *Chapter 6*, you are liable to come across individuals from all walks of life. You will find as much variety in dress, thinking and behaviour as there are fashions, ranging from the formal and sophisticated to the absolutely informal.

Equally, you will find their premises very different.

Some will present a 'brass plaque' image, working in a clinic with a receptionist and brisk efficiency, while others will see you in their living room surrounded by plants and domestic clutter.

Remember, though, that while image may be some indication of status, it is little guarantee of ability. You are as likely to find a therapist of quality working from home as in a formal clinic.

Some characteristics, though, and probably the most important ones, are common to all natural therapists:

- They will give you far more time than you are used to with a family doctor. An initial consultation will rarely last less than an hour, and is often longer. They will ask you all about yourself so they can form a proper understanding of what makes you tick and what may be the fundamental cause(s) of your problem.

- You will have to pay for any remedies they prescribe, and they may well sell you these from their own stocks. They will also charge you for their time – though many therapists offer reduced fees for deserving cases or for people who genuinely cannot afford the full fee.

## Sensible precautions

- Be sceptical of anyone who 'guarantees' you a cure. No one (not even doctors) can do that.
- Query any attempt to book you in for a course of treatment. Your response to any natural therapy is highly individual. Of course, if the practice is a busy one, booking ahead for one or two sessions might be sensible. You should be able to cancel without penalty any sessions which prove unnecessary (but remember to give at least 24 hours' notice: some practitioners will charge you if you don't give enough notice).

- No ethical therapist will ask for fees in advance of treatment unless for special tests or medicines – and even this is unusual. If you are asked for 'down payments' of any sort, ask exactly what they are for. If you don't like the reasons, don't pay.

- Be wary if you are not asked about your existing medication and try to give precise answers when you are asked. Be especially wary if the therapist tells you to stop or change any medically prescribed drug without talking to your doctor first. (A responsible doctor should also be happy to discuss you and your medication with a therapist.)

- Note the quality of the therapist's touch if you choose any of the relaxation or manipulation techniques such as massage, aromatherapy or osteopathy. It should never be lingering or suggestive. If, for any reason, the therapist wants to touch you on the breasts or genitals, your permission should be sought first.

- If the practitioner is of the opposite sex you are entitled to have someone of your choice in the room at the same time. Be immediately suspicious if this is not allowed. Ethical therapists will not refuse this sort of request, and if they do, it is probably best to have nothing more to do with them.

## What to do if things go wrong

A practitioner is in a position of trust, and is charged with a duty of care to you at all times. It does not mean you are 'entitled' to a 'cure' just because you've paid for treatment, but if you feel you are being treated unfairly, incompetently or unethically, you have several options:

- Tackle the matter at the source of the problem, with your practitioner, either verbally or in writing.

- If he or she works in a place such as a clinic, health farm or sports centre, tell the management. They also have a duty to protect the public and should treat complaints seriously and discreetly.
- Contact the practitioner's professional organization. It should have an independent panel that investigates complaints fully and disciplines its members.
- If the offence committed is a criminal one report it to the police (but be prepared for the problem of proving one person's word against another's).
- If you feel compensation is due see a lawyer for advice.

Short of a public court case, the worst thing for a truly incompetent or unethical practitioner is bad publicity. Tell everyone about your experiences. People only need to hear the same sort of comments from a few different sources and the practitioner will probably sink without trace. Before you do so, though, try the other measures first and give yourself time to consider things calmly. Vengeance is not very healing.

*A word of warning* Don't make malicious allegations without good reason. Such actions are themselves a criminal offence in most countries and you could end up in more trouble than the practitioner.

## Summary

The reality is that there are few crooks or charlatans in natural therapy. Despite the myth, there is little real money in it unless the therapist is very busy – and the chances are high that a busy therapist is a good one. Remember that no one can know everything and no specialist qualified in any field has to get 100 per cent in the exams to be able to practise. Perfection is an ideal, not a reality, and to err is human.

It is very much for this reason that taking control of your own health is perhaps the single most important lesson underlying this book. Taking control means taking responsibility for the choices you make, and this is one of the most significant factors in successful treatment.

No one but you can decide on a practitioner and no one but you can determine if that practitioner is any good or not. You will know this very easily, and probably very quickly, by the way you feel about the person and the therapy, and by whether or not you get any better.

If you are not happy, the decision is yours whether to stay or move on – and continue moving until you find the right therapist for you. Don't despair if you don't find the right person first time. There is almost bound to be the right person for you somewhere and your determination to get well is the best resource you have for finding that person.

Above all, bear in mind that many people who have taken this route before you have not only been helped beyond their most optimistic dreams, but have also found a close and trusted helper who will assist in times of trouble – and who may even become a friend for life.

# Useful organizations

*The following listing of organizations is for information only and does not imply any endorsement, nor do the organizations listed necessarily agree with the views expressed in this book.*

## INTERNATIONAL

**International Federation of Multiple Sclerosis Societies**
10 Heddon Street
London W1R 7JL, UK.
Tel 0171 734 9120
Fax 0171 287 2587

**International Federation of Practitioners of Natural Therapeutics**
10 Copse Close
Sheet
Petersfield
Hampshire GU31 4DL, UK.
Tel 01730 266790
Fax 01730 260058

**Persons with MS International**
*see* International Federation of MS Societies

## AUSTRALASIA

**Australian Natural Therapists Association**
PO Box 308
Melrose Park
South Australia 5039.
Tel 618 297 9533
Fax 618 297 0003

**Australian Traditional Medicine Society**
PO Box 442 *or*
Suite 3, First Floor,
120 Blaxland Road
Ryde
New South Wales 2112
Australia.
Tel 612 808 2825
Fax 612 809 7570

**MS Society of New Zealand**
7th Floor, Rossmore House
123 Molesworth Street
PO Box 2627
Wellington
New Zealand.
Tel 644 499 4677
Fax 644 499 4675

**National MS Society of Australia**
Private Bag Q1000
QVB Post Office
Sydney
New South Wales 2000
Australia.
Tel 612 287 2929
Fax 612 287 2987

**New Zealand Natural Health Practitioners Accreditation Board**
PO Box 37–491
Auckland, New Zealand.
Tel 9 625 9966
*Supported by 15 therapy organizations.*

## NORTH AMERICA

**American Academy of Medical Preventics**
6151 West Century Boulevard, Suite 1114
Los Angeles
California 90045, USA.
Tel 213 645 5350

**American Association of Naturopathic Physicians**
2800 East Madison Street, Suite 200
Seattle
Washington 98112, USA
*or*
PO Box 20386
Seattle
Washington 98102, USA.
Tel 206 323 7610
Fax 206 323 7612

**American Holistic Medical Association**
4101 Lake Boone Trail, Suite 201
Raleigh
North Carolina 27607, USA.
Tel 919 787 5146
Fax 919 787 4916

**Canadian Holistic Medical Association**
700 Bay Street
PO Box 101, Suite 604
Toronto
Ontario M5G 1Z6, Canada.
Tel 416 599 0447

**International Biooxydative Medicine Foundation**
PO Box 13205
Oklahoma City
Oklahoma 73113, USA.
Fax 405 634 0375
*For information on treatment by intravenous $H_2O_2$.*

**MS Society of Canada**
250 Bloor St East, Suite 820
Toronto
Ontario M4W 3P9, Canada.
Tel 416 922 6065
Fax 416 922 7538

**National Multiple Sclerosis Society**
205 East 42 Street
New York
New York 10017 5700, USA.
Tel 212 986 3420
Fax 212 986 7981

## SOUTHERN AFRICA

**MS Society of Zimbabwe**
PO Box 8214
Causeway
Harare
Zimbabwe.
Tel 263 796 957

South African Homoeopaths,
Chiropractors & Allied
Professions Board
PO Box 17055
0027 Groenkloof
South Africa.
Tel 1246 6455

South African National MS
Society
295 Villiers Road, Walmer
Port Elizabeth 6070
South Africa.
Tel/fax 4151 2900

## UK AND EIRE

British Association for
Counselling
1 Regent Place
Rugby
Warwicks CV21 2PJ, UK.
Tel 01788 578328/9

British Complementary
Medicine Association
39 Prestbury Road
Pitville
Cheltenham
Gloucestershire GL52 2PT, UK.
Tel 01242 226770
Fax 01242 226778

British Holistic Medical
Association
Trust House
Royal Shrewsbury Hospital
South
Shrewsbury
Shropshire SY3 8XF, UK.
Tel 01743 261155
Fax 01743 3536373

Council for Complementary &
Alternative Medicine
179 Gloucester Place
London NW1 6DX, UK.
Tel 0171 724 9103
Fax 0171 724 5330

Disability Alliance
Universal House
Wentworth Street
London E1 7SA, UK.
Tel 0171 247 8776
*Benefits and rights enquiries hotline
0171 247 8763 (Mon/Wed 2–4pm,
Fri 10.30–12.30).*

Disabled Living Foundation
380-384 Harrow Road
London W9 2HU, UK.
Tel 0171 289 6111
Fax 0171 266 2922

Federation of Multiple Sclerosis
Therapy Centres
Unit 4
Murdock Road
Bedford MK41 7PD, UK.
Tel 01234 325781
*A network of 67 self-governing local
patient support centres covering
Great Britain and Eire set up in
1993.*

Institute for Complementary
Medicine
PO Box 194
London SE16 1QZ, UK.
Tel 0171 237 5165
Fax 0171 237 5175

**Multiple Sclerosis Resource Centre**
4a Chapel Hill
Stansted
Essex CM24 8AG, UK.
Tel 01279 817101
Fax 01279 647179

**Multiple Sclerosis Society of Great Britain & Northern Ireland**
25 Effie Road
London SW6 1YZ, UK.
Tel 0171 610 7171
Fax 0171 736 9861

*Helpline (Mon – Fri, 10am – 4pm)*
*Tel 0171 371 8000*

**Multiple Sclerosis Society of Ireland**
2 Sandymount Green
Dublin 4
Eire.
Tel 0126 94599
Fax 0126 93746

**Multiple Sclerosis Training, Education & Research Trust (MUSTER)**
MUSTER Communications
Unit 67
49 Effra Road
London SW2 IBZ , UK.
Tel 0171 738 3288
Fax 0171 738 6212
*MUSTER was set up in 1994 in succession to Action & Research in Multiple Sclerosis (ARMS).*

**MS Under Pressure (Susie Cornell)**
PO Box 1270
Chelmsford
Essex CM2 6BQ, UK.
Tel 01245 268098
Fax 01245 252280

**Oxygen Therapies Information Centre**
13 Albert Road
Retford
Notts DN22 6JD, UK.
Tel 01777 710292

**The British Trust for the Myelin Project**
Craigievar House
77 Craigmount Brae
Edinburgh EH12 8XF
Scotland.
Tel 0131 339 1316
Fax 0131 317 1316

**Yoga for Health Foundation**
Ickwell Bury
Biggleswade
Bedfordshire SG18 9EF, UK.
Tel 01767 627271

# APPENDIX B

# Useful further reading

*Acupressure for Common Ailments*, Chris Jarmey and John Tindall (Gaia Books, UK, 1991)

*Acupuncture*, George Lewith (Thorsons, UK, 1982)

*Coping with MS*, Cynthia Benz (Macdonald-Optima, UK, 1988)

*Family Guide to Alternative Medicine*, ed Patrick Pietroni (Reader's Digest Association, UK/USA, 1991)

*Healing Nutrients*, Patrick Quillen (Contemporary Books, USA/Beaverbooks, Canada, 1987, Penguin, UK, 1989)

*Illustrated Encyclopaedia of Essential Oils*, Julia Lawless (Element Books, UK/USA, 1995)

*Life, Health and Longevity*, Kenneth Seaton (Scientific Hygiene, USA, 1994)

*Maximising Your Health in MS*, D Frankel and R Buxbaum (National MS Society, USA, 1982)

*MS Special Diet Cookbook*, Geraldine Fitzgerald and Fenella Briscoe (Harper/Collins, UK, 1989)

*Multiple Sclerosis: A Guide for Patients and their Families*, L C Scheinberg (National MS Society, USA)

*Multiple Sclerosis – The Facts*, W B Matthews (Oxford University Press, UK, 1993)

*Multiple Sclerosis: The Self-Help Guide*, Judy Graham (Thorsons, UK, 1992)

*Prescription for Nutritional Healing*, James and Phyllis Balch (Avery Press, USA, 1990)

*Raw Energy*, Leslie & Susannah Kenton (Arrow Books, UK, 1985)

*The Art of Reflexology*, Inge Dougans and Suzanne Ellis (Element Books, UK/USA, 1992)

*The Family Guide to Homoeopathy*, Andrew Lockie (Hamish Hamilton, UK, 1990)

*The New Holistic Herbal*, David Hoffman (Element Books, UK/USA, 1990/92)

*Yoga for the Disabled*, Howard Kent (Thorsons, UK, 1985)

*You Can Heal Your Life*, Louise Hay (Eden Grove, USA, 1988)

# Index